Be Healthy

Be Healthy

simple guidelines for lifelong well-being

Stories from the United States and Africa

Ed Dodge, MD, MPH

FOUNDATION FOR HEALTHY AFRICA

SAN ANTONIO, TEXAS

Endorsements

"Dr. Dodge has provided a succinct road map for long-lived vigor and true quality of life. It is backed up by scientific evidence, practical experience, and a lifetime of wisdom."

Michelle Holmes, MD, MPH, Dr.PH.
Associate Professor, Dept. of Epidemiology
Harvard School of Public Health

"Dr. Dodge's book, *Be Healthy*, is written to inspire and it does so with honesty and style. Through use of personal experience and practical knowledge, Dr. Dodge moves the reader from complacency to action. The end result is a new view of health that is hard to ignore. The book's guidelines provide both map and compass to guide the reader along a path of better physical, emotional, and spiritual health. In nonjudgmental language, Dr. Dodge inspires the reader to choose wellness in a way that is personalized and effective."

David M. Deci, M.D.
Associate Professor and Director
Office of Medical Student Education
Department of Family Medicine
University of Wisconsin

"*Be Healthy* is easy to read, provides the right amount and kind of information, has a comprehensive view of the topic, provides the science for its claims, and uses personal cases to inspire and bring the concepts into life. I read it to my great inspiration and profit."

Arne Hassing, Ph.D.
Retired Professor of Comparative Cultural Studies

"*Be Healthy* is very powerful. It empowers the reader to take action / responsibility for their own health. In my experience it is the first book to deal with most of the risk factors on chronic- non-communicable diseases (NCDs) in a comprehensive manner. The life experience in the book further enhances the belief that it is possible to reverse the growing problem of NCDs when individuals modify their behaviors or lifestyles."

Clemencia Bakasa
Deputy Minister of Health
Office of Noncommunicable Diseases
Zimbabwe

"I've stopped counting all the invaluable things I learned in this power-packed book. Dr. Dodge doesn't just tell us how to live a healthy life—lots of books do that; Dr. Dodge explains why in simple clear language and provides the research to back it up. His explanation of the acid-alkaline impact of meat and dairy vs plant-based foods alone will change your diet forever. With *Be Healthy* on my bookshelf, I do not think I need another book on health."

Janet Conner, *Writing Down Your Soul, My Soul Pages, The Lotus and The Lily*

"*Be Healthy* is an eye-opener and a wake-up call. Real change starts with clarity—a clear understanding, a clear mindset and a clear target. This book delivers all three. Dr. Dodge shows us clearly that we all have powerful choices to make. This is one of the great things about this book—he tells us what he knows and how he actually does it! Real stuff. Wherever you are—sick or well, knowledgeable or new to health, we can all benefit from Dr. Dodge's experience of the power of lifestyle. His guidance makes this book a winner."

Mike Kinnaird, author of *The Happy Guide*

"Ed Dodge's *Be Healthy* is a book everyone interested in living a healthier, more meaningful, life will want to read. Eminently practical, yet research based, Dr. Dodge presents the reader with suggestions that anyone can adopt in their own daily lives, to achieve a healthier, more meaningful life. What's more, he makes it clear that adopting these practices need not require deprivation—quite the contrary—they promise to also add to the joy and quality of life."

Frederick Kirschenmann, author of *Cultivating an Ecological Conscience: Essays From a Farmer Philosopher*

Be Healthy: Simple Guidelines for Lifelong Well-being
Copyright © Edward Dodge 2014

Published by Foundation for Healthy Africa
P.O. Box 592691
San Antonio, TX 78258
ThePowerofLifestyle.com

ISBN: 978-0-9912365-1-0
eISBN: 978-0-9912365-0-3

Project Development/Editor: Jo Ann Deck
Book Cover, Design, Typesetting: Ja-lene Clark, GatherInsight.com
Cover Art: Istock
Chapter Opening Art: "Reflection Joy" painting by Bernard Ndichu Njuguna of Kenya
Additional Photo Credits:
Innocent Chamusingareve: photo by Privilege Mutande
Randall Dodge: photo by Amber Berry
Hellen Dziwa: photo by Davidson Dziwa
Kudzayi Mukosera: photo by Chishamiso Mukosera
Balwani C. Mbakaya: photo by Temwani Mbakaya

Medical Disclaimer: This book and its contents are not intended to be a substitute for medical advice from a physician. A physician should be consulted if you have any health concerns or symptoms that may require diagnosis or medical attention.

PRINTED IN THE USA

Dedication

To my readers: This book was written for you.

Contents

Introduction 12

CHAPTER ONE: Ed's Story 15

CHAPTER TWO: Randall's Story 25

CHAPTER THREE: Your Story 39

THE POWER OF LIFESTYLE

CHAPTER FOUR: Eat Wholesome Foods Abundantly 46

CHAPTER FIVE: Minimize Sabotaging Foods! 51

CHAPTER SIX: Foods with a Question Mark 63

CHAPTER SEVEN: Create Healthy Meals 73

CHAPTER EIGHT: The Dreadful "Sitting Disease" 92

CHAPTER NINE: The Awesome Benefits of

Physical Activity 98

CHAPTER TEN: A Simple Plan to Be Physically Active 108

CHAPTER ELEVEN: Personal and Mental Hygiene 120

CHAPTER TWELVE: Good Environmental Hygiene 138

CHAPTER THIRTEEN: Caring Relationships 154

CHAPTER FOURTEEN: Health and Well-Being 167

CHAPTER FIFTEEN: The Power of Lifestyle 182

LIFESTYLE STORIES FROM AFRICA

CHAPTER SIXTEEN: Mbakaya's Story   203

CHAPTER SEVENTEEN: Hellen's Story   209

CHAPTER EIGHTEEN: Innocent's Story   217

CHAPTER NINETEEN: Kudzayi's Story   222

Epilogue   232

APPENDIX A: Chemicals in Our Environment   235

APPENDIX B: The Wellness Toolkit —

               Practicing the Power of Lifestyle   245

About Dr. Ed Dodge   250

The Foundation for Healthy Africa   252

Acknowledgments

Thanks first of all to my wife Carol, who generously gave me all the time and space I needed to work on this project. This was no small gift. I could not have written this book without it. But that is not her only contribution. She is enthusiastic about healthful eating, and we work together on preparing healthy meals. Her help and her support in all aspects of our lifestyle is invaluable!

Thanks to my son and contributing author, Randall, who tells his story so effectively early in this book, and who contributed significantly to several other chapters. Thanks also to his wife, Colleen. They're a delightful couple.

Thanks to my MPH student authors: Balwani-Mbakaya Chingatichifwe, Hellen Dziwa, Innocent Chamusingarevi and Kudzayi Mukosera. They absorbed the importance and value of lifestyle teachings through their Masters of Public Health classes at Africa University, applied them to their own lives, and now share their own stories in Chapters 17-20. Thanks also to all my other students at Africa University. They are my teachers as well as my students, and we have a good time learning together.

Thanks to my colleagues at Africa University for their friendship and their warm support of my teaching about the power of lifestyle.

Thanks to my son Jeff and his wife Tammi, and my daughter Amy and her husband Paul, for their helpful suggestions, their good humor about lifestyle, and the way they and their families meet and handle life's exigencies so well.

Thanks to my sister, Lois Stewart, for her helpful review of my manuscript. Thanks also to everyone in my extended family for being supportive of my health-oriented teachings and writings.

Thanks to the early reviewers of my manuscript for giving me their valuable time and suggestions.

Thanks to Janet Conner for teaching me the value of soulful journaling in her powerful workshop on this subject.

Thanks to the many pioneers (too many to name) in the health arena who have shown the power of lifestyle so effectively as they plowed new ground in this field. Happily, their ranks continue to grow dramatically.

Thanks to my many teachers and professors at Taylor University, the Indiana University School of Medicine, and the Johns Hopkins School of Hygiene and Public Health. They laid a foundation on which I could continue to build with confidence in my lifelong pursuit of knowledge and wisdom.

Thanks to my parents, Ralph and Eunice Dodge (now deceased,) who were my first indelible teachers and models of healthy living.

Thanks to Jo Ann Deck, my editor and literary agent, who contributed immeasurably to this book with her incisive questions and superb editing. Jo Ann has become a friend, and I'm deeply grateful to her for her continuing faith in the worth of this book through its many metamorphoses.

Thanks to Cheryl Harrison, webmaster and editor of my Wellness Newsletter, for her helpful insights and suggestions about publishing eBooks. Cheryl is a good friend and I greatly value her suggestions.

Thanks to Ja-lene Clark from GatherInsight.com for her invaluable help as layout editor for this book. Ja-lene pulled everything together beautifully in creating this book. Thank you, Ja-lene!

Finally, thanks to the countless people who have contributed to teaching me about what is valuable in life, and to you, our readers, for your willingness and courage to explore the power of lifestyle.

Introduction

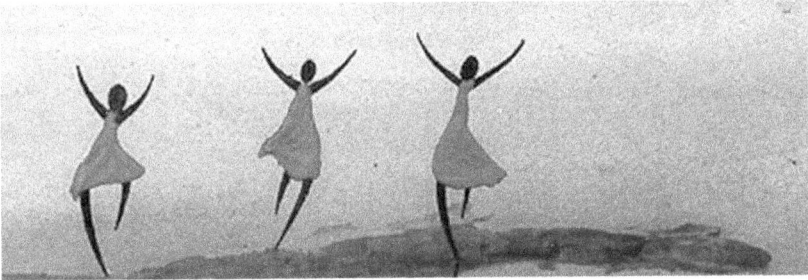

You can enjoy excellent health in youth and throughout life as you get older. That's the message of this book.

Unfortunately, many people experience declining health or have serious health issues by the time they reach middle age. More often than not, this doesn't have to be the case. Science tells us that up to 80 percent of serious health problems such as heart disease, hypertension or type 2 diabetes can be prevented. The key to prevention is a healthy lifestyle.

There is general agreement on the principles of healthy living. While there may be a few differences of opinion on details of a healthy lifestyle, most people recognize the important underlying principles: healthy eating, healthy exercise, good hygiene, and a healthy emotional life.

The power of lifestyle to nurture good health is remarkable. Recognizing this, lifestyle initiatives have been launched in the past decade by many leading medical organizations. These include Harvard University's Institute of Lifestyle Medicine, the Cleveland Clinic's Wellness Institute, Northwestern University's Center for Lifestyle Medicine and many others.

The American, Australian, and European Colleges of Lifestyle Medicine were also established in the past ten years.

Lifestyle medicine is in the forefront of preventing and treating the underlying causes of our most serious health problems. We apply this cutting-edge approach to better health in this book. Its life prescriptions are easy to understand. If followed faithfully, they lead to improved health and well-being. Unhappily, consistent application turns out to be a stumbling block for many of us. We know what to do for the sake of good health, and yet we often falter or fail to do what's best for us.

I've grappled with this paradox in my own life. A brief story of my life is found in chapter one. I tell this story at the outset to let you know who I am. As I have struggled with a variety of issues, my understanding of how to cope with them has grown through the years.

As a family physician, I've helped many people deal with health issues. I'm now retired from family practice, but I continue to teach healthy lifestyle practices in my classes and workshops. I can't be your doctor, but as you read this book, please know that I'm familiar with both the pitfalls and the joys of striving for a healthy lifestyle. I'm on your side to encourage you to be your best, even through the toughest of times.

In this book we deal with health challenges realistically, but also optimistically. Although this is not an academic tome, it is well supported by science. Designed as a book of practical information, it offers guidance to anyone wishing to achieve better health. Make this book a useful health tool. You can make a difference in your own life!

CHAPTER ONE

Ed's Story

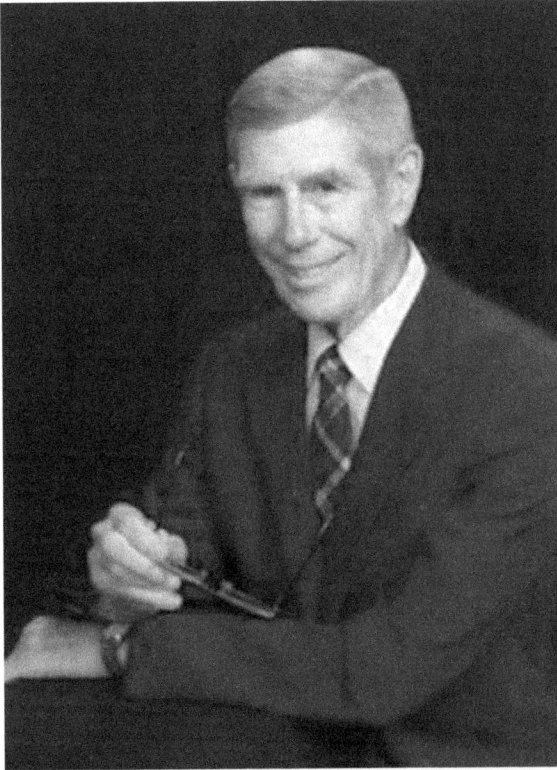

I grew up in Angola, Africa, arriving as a baby with my missionary parents in 1936. During my pre-teen years, we lived in the Dembos region, a forested highland area of northern Angola that was still primitive. We lived on Dad's garden produce, including corn, peas, beans, greens, beets, carrots, sweet potatoes and various kinds of squash. Having grown up on a farm, gardening was his hobby, and he always had a great garden wherever we lived. We also had a few goats and some chickens that provided us with occasional meat and eggs.

Wild game was plentiful and it supplied some of our meat. Dad took one day off a month to go hunting, taking me with him after I turned twelve. He usually got a bushbuck or an African buffalo, and I even shot a buffalo on our final hunt. We had fresh or dried meat with some of our meals. With no access to processed foods, our diet was simple, but truly healthy.

Our home in the Dembos area was a four-room mud and stick house, similar to indigenous homes, but a bit larger than most of them. The kitchen, shower and storage rooms were separate from the living area, and we had an outhouse out back. Our water was carried from a spring about a mile away. The "shower" was a bucket on a simple pulley arrangement. When I took a "shower," I simply tipped the bucket to rinse off the suds.

The main room in the house was not large, but it served multiple purposes. A table with six chairs sat in the middle, and we ate our meals there. The same table served as a study table for us home-schooled kids, and it was a work table for my parents in the evenings. Finally, the room was our living-room when we had occasional visiting guests.

We had no electricity. Our stove was wood-burning, which was why the kitchen was separate from the main house. We had a kerosene refrigerator that worked well when we had kerosene. We also used kerosene lamps for the main room. As a rule, we went to bed early because the lighting was not great. Of course, we also got up early.

We returned to the States in 1950. Dad had been appointed Foreign Division Secretary of the Methodist Board of Missions for its work throughout Europe and Africa. The Board of Missions office was in New York. We rented a home in Ridgewood, New Jersey so Dad could commute to New York City by train. I started 10th grade in Ridgewood High School. Suffering from reverse culture shock, I was pretty much of a loner in high school, but I graduated in 1953.

Taylor University, a small interdenominational college in Upland, Indiana, was perfect for me. Missionary kids were common there. I felt understood, made friends, and began to feel at home in the United States. I majored in biology, a subject I loved, with the idea of becoming a biology teacher. However, in my junior year I decided to switch to a pre-med course. Since I had not taken any chemistry or physics, it took five years for me to finish my pre-med requirements.

I entered Indiana University School of Medicine in 1958, graduating with honors in 1962. In the meantime, having married Nancy DeLay, my college sweetheart from Taylor, our little family began to grow. Randy was born while I was in medical school, and Jeffrey was born during my internship at Los Angeles County General Hospital. Internship was tough for us as a family, but it was a year of professional growth for me. With 3,600 beds, Los Angeles County General Hospital was one of the largest in the USA. Caring for patients with a wide range of diseases and trauma, I learned a great deal of practical, hands-on medicine.

Interns practically lived at the hospital, working on call every second or third night. The hospital offered a midnight meal for staff on duty. Free meals were one of the few perks for interns, so we took advantage of every meal possible. I ate most of my meals there, including the midnight meal when I was on call. Within six months I had gained 15 pounds and my hospital whites had become too tight. I had to lose weight or get new uniforms which we couldn't afford. By cutting out desserts and the midnight meal, I succeeded in returning to my normal weight.

After completing my medical and public health training (MD in 1962 and MPH in 1967), I worked in Ethiopia for two years. Nancy and our three young children went with me. Located in the Horn of Africa, Ethiopia is a mountainous country with extensive central plateaus where most of the people live. I taught at the Public Health College in Gondar and supervised student interns who staffed the rural Training Health Centers.

As a result of my work at the Training Health Centers, I learned much about rural Ethiopian lifestyles. Rural Ethiopians of that era were lean and almost entirely free of our Western diseases. Major health problems included childhood malnutrition as well as classic infectious and parasitic diseases. People were very active, walking miles a day at their work, to fetch water from the nearest spring or river, or go to market on market days. If a school was available, children would walk miles for any educational opportunity.

Their diet was simple, consisting of injera and wat for most of their meals. Injera is a pancake-like sour bread made from tef, the predominant grain in Ethiopia. Wat is the spicy sauce eaten with injera. Vegetable-based, it may be enriched with egg, chicken, or mutton on feast days. It is often flavored with traditional hot beriberi sauce. The chickens were all free-range, and the sheep were all grazing animals. No processed foods were available in rural villages at that time.

In the town of Gondar, where we lived, it was possible to buy some canned goods and a few other minimally processed foods, but we didn't get many of them. We had a garden that produced some vegetables and fruit. A small flock of chickens at the back of our compound kept us supplied with eggs. There was a great vegetable farm near town, so we had an abundant source of fresh vegetables.

I had injera and wat frequently at the Training Centers, and my family also learned to like it. The kids loved it, and we had it at home once or twice a week. We ate chicken occasionally. Red meat was not easily available, and we rarely ate it.

We had no television. On my free weekends, we often took family hikes to explore various parts of the countryside around us. Gondar had been the capital of Ethiopia from the mid-1600s to the mid-1800s. Even though many of the castles of that era are now in ruins, they are reminders of Gondar's grand heritage. There were also ruins of various castles and churches in the surrounding countryside, and we sometimes went to see one of them, or simply to enjoy the beauty of the countryside.

We did a lot of this, particularly during our second year when we had become more familiar with the area. Our treks usually lasted for two or three hours. Randy was nine, Jeff was six, and Amy had just turned two. We stopped frequently to look at the sights around us, and I carried Amy when she got tired. Though our pace was slow, we did lots of walking. In retrospect, those family hikes were wonderful times of bonding for all of us.

Back in the States, I worked for the Frontier Nursing Service in the mountains of Eastern Kentucky for a year and a half. I was one of two doctors staffing the general clinic and the small 16-bed hospital. Although the differences between it and the enormous Los Angeles County General Hospital were like night and day, it was also a challenging experience. I was on call every other night, and with no specialist located closer than an hour or two away, we had to be very resourceful.

We also backed up six nursing clinics, staffed by Nurse-Midwives, located in remote mountain hamlets. These licensed Nurse-Midwives were well trained, but the Frontier Nursing Service felt an urgent need for Family Nurse-practitioners. Part of my work was to help teach in one of the first Family Nurse-Practitioner training programs in the country.

Nancy and the children enjoyed our life there, but after a year and a half I took a position as the Director of the two-county Citrus-Levy Health Department in Central Florida. Having grown up in St. Petersburg, Nancy was familiar with that area. We felt it would be a good location to put down roots as a family.

I enjoyed my work as the Director of a small local Health Department, but in 1975 I was invited to join a family practice group in Inverness. I worked as a member of the group for the next 21 years. I loved my work as a family physician. Helping individuals and families with health issues was rewarding work, and I developed friendships with many people in the area, especially in the health field.

The work was demanding, both because of the nature of medical care and because physicians were in short supply. I spent long hours in my office and then additional hours at our local hospital to ensure good care for my patients. Though our hospital was not especially large, it was a good community hospital with a dedicated medical and nursing staff. I valued the years I spent there, giving my best for my patients and community.

In 1991, Nancy received devastating news. A routine Pap test revealed evidence of cancer. Follow-up testing at the University of Florida confirmed an unusual tubo-ovarian cancer. Nancy proceeded to have major surgery, and then a rigorous course of chemotherapy because of the finding of multiple metastases at the time of surgery. During this time Nancy wished to stop eating red meat, and we decided to become semi-vegetarian. After completion of her chemotherapy she was much better, and we had high hopes for a full recovery.

Unfortunately, her cancer recurred. A second course of chemotherapy was less successful. In 1996 she had metastases to her brain requiring emergency brain surgery followed by radiation to the brain. I took an early retirement at that point to help care for her at home. It was one of the best decisions I ever made. The next two years were bittersweet. In spite of her illness, we were able to spend much good quality time together. Still, as her condition deteriorated, it was wrenching. Nancy taught me much about coping with both life and death.

I went to a spiritual retreat a few months after her death, looking for some re-direction. I had been out of medical practice for three years, and at age 63, I thought I was a bit too old to begin the rigors of building a new medical practice. I considered becoming more involved in church work, and the retreat strengthened this idea.

The retreat also pointed me in an unexpected direction. I met a lady there named Carol Fitzgerald from San Antonio Texas. We struck up a friendship that developed into a long-distance courtship, and we got married in December 1999.

In 2004 I joined a Volunteer-in-Mission (VIM) team going to work on a church-related community development project in Zimbabwe for two weeks. I made many friends and found the experience so rewarding that I returned again in 2007 and 2009. At that time I met Dr. Peter Fasan, Dean of the Faculty of Health Sciences at Africa University. He invited me to consider doing some short-term teaching the next year.

After going over this possibility with Carol and praying for guidance, I accepted Dr. Fasan's invitation. Carol and I moved to San Antonio where she had a supportive network, and in August 2010 I began serving as a Visiting Adjunct Professor of Non-communicable Diseases in the public health program at Africa University. I have taught this subject at both the undergraduate and Master of Public Health levels for one semester each year since then.

To say that I've enjoyed this experience is an understatement. Working with students and colleagues in the Faculty of Health Sciences has been a joy, and the entire experience of working and teaching in Africa has been a dream come true. It brings me full circle from having been cradled in the heart of Africa to celebrating my golden years there. In between, it has been my great privilege to work toward better health in both Africa and America.

I have been remarkably blessed to have a bird's eye view of the health field from every possible vantage. I saw the devastating impact of malaria and other communicable diseases all around me as a child. In medical school I learned the skills of good patient care. At the Johns Hopkins School of Public Health, I learned the importance of understanding and treating disease on a population-wide basis. During my career, I have worked in the front lines of both public health and individual patient care. I've taken part in health care from multiple perspectives: private physician, public health administrator, patient, patient advocate, and teacher. In all of this, I've absorbed many life lessons that have been both humbling and exhilarating.

One of the major lessons I've learned is that health vitality is an inner gift—one that each of us can nurture better than anyone else. Medical professionals are often given credit for being healers, and the work they do can be very important in restoring health. Yet, they are not the real healers. French physician Ambroise Paré, often called the father of surgery, put it best when he said, "I only put in the stitches. God does the healing." The same principle applies for all of medicine.

My purpose in writing this book is to share what I've learned through the years about what each of us can do to nurture our own vitality. Your health power is greater than you realize. I hope this book helps you grasp this as you learn about tips, techniques and habits that can enhance your health, physically, mentally, emotionally and spiritually. Let your own magnificence shine!

CHAPTER TWO

Randall's Story

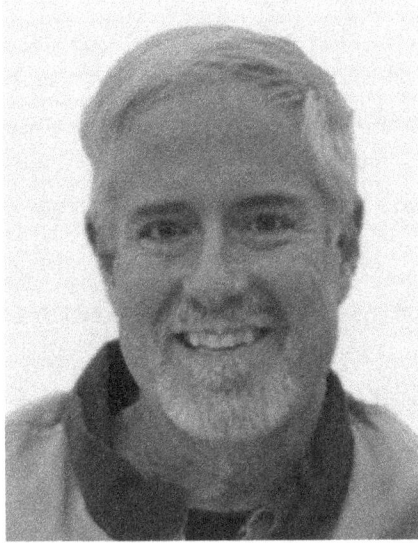

"A new report on obesity in this country is out tonight with some sobering stats. In 1995, not a single state in the country had an obesity rate above 20 percent of the population. Now all the states but one do and Colorado, the only one, is barely hanging on with 19.8 percent of its residents considered obese."

Juan Williams, NBC Nightly News (7/7/2011)

Hi, my name is Randall and I am the eldest son of Dr. Ed Dodge. I am not a health care professional but I am concerned about declining health issues in the United States. So I have learned and applied a few lessons about improving my own health. I do not want to participate any longer in the obesity epidemic that is plaguing this country.

As I write this, I am in my fifties and within a "normal" weight range for my height (BMI=24). My fitness and nutrition levels reveal good evidence of health. But this was not always the case. After decades of being obese and out of shape, I recently lost weight and made a commitment to live a healthier lifestyle. Dad (Ed) has asked me to share my story with you and I am delighted to do so. In addition, I will share some application tips and suggestions that I have found helpful along the way. Feel free to try any or all of these suggestions and use the ones that work for you. If you find something else that works better for you, please let me know. You won't hurt my feelings a bit if you tell me you found an even better way to get healthier!

Before I share my personal health journey, let me first share some "insider information" about Dad. Who can better attest to the "real" Dr. Ed Dodge than one of his own family members? Not everyone who writes about health has the educational credentials, the professional experience and the history of personal application to earn your trust. Dad has all three. His credentials, experience and lifestyle are consistent. Dad walks the talk and he has done so for a long, long time. Healthy living has been his lifelong focus. From my earliest memories, Dad has always enjoyed good health that is based on sound nutrition principles, regular exercise, clean living, committed relationships, and moderation in all things.

I'm not sure what first sparked Dad's fire for healthy living. Maybe it happened while he was growing up in Africa and experiencing firsthand the community benefits of a largely plant-based diet. This love for fresh vegetables and fruits was only reinforced by his father (my grandfather) who was an avid gardener. Maybe Dad's lifelong passion for healthy living was sparked by walking everywhere he wanted to go in a rural African community in which pedestrian travel was considered the normal way for everyone to get around. Or perhaps it was the interpersonal relationships Dad developed early in life with family and friends without the influence of modern technology. Growing their own food, preparing it for family meals and cleaning up together were all part of forming deeper relationships than are typically afforded in a Western, convenience-centered culture.

For his professional training, Dad studied medicine at Indiana University and then public health at Johns Hopkins University. His first-class medical education gave him the tools to better understand the roots of healthy living. And while he was a top-notch family physician, Dad was never conceited about his role as a medical doctor. He told each of his patients that they exercised more influence over their own health through their daily decisions than he could through periodic checkups. And if they would practice healthy living principles, the results would be evident for all to see.

To prove his point, Dad modeled the joys of healthy living in his private life. Throughout my childhood, healthy, whole foods were served at every meal in our family home. During the aerobic running movement of the 1970's, Dad was up before dawn to go jogging each weekday morning. With all of his three kids on the high school tennis team, Dad installed a court in the back yard and maintained weekly tennis matches with friends on weekends. In addition to jogging and tennis, other activities like cycling, hiking, canoeing and swimming were all part of Dad's lifelong fitness program.

The result was that I never saw Dad's weight fluctuate by more than a few pounds. He has always been fit and trim, ready to engage with his children and now grandchildren in whatever activities they ask him to join. And now when most people are retired, Dad's lifestyle exemplifies the joys and benefits of consistent healthy living. He travels the world, teaching in colleges and universities, hosting radio programs and writing about the joys of healthy living. He is absolutely convinced that everyone can experience these joys and benefits for themselves. And he has convinced me that I can too. But as a bit of a slow learner or perhaps just stubborn son, I took more convincing than most. Here is my story.

As already mentioned, I enjoyed sports in school, lettering four years on the varsity tennis team. I also enjoyed competitive canoe racing and bicycle touring. The summer after I graduated from college I rode my bicycle across the United States from the Pacific to the Atlantic Ocean and then the next summer, I did it again.

To a casual observer, I looked healthy in my early twenties. I was fit and had an athletic build. But there was a hidden time bomb about to go off, even if ever so gradually. You see, I wasn't committed to lifelong, daily exercise and I never fully bought into the healthy nutrition principles I had observed as a child. Oh sure, I enjoyed a good salad, so long as it was just a side salad with pizza or cheeseburgers and followed by something sweet like ice cream or cookies or both.

Food was fuel for my activities but in times of stress it became a source of comfort. I was especially fond of foods processed from flour or sugar or both. What I didn't know was that I was developing an addiction to the chemicals produced in my body when I flooded my bloodstream with these refined carbohydrates. And the long-term effect was so gradual that it was almost imperceptible. Kind of like the proverbial frog that won't jump out of the saucepan as the water temperature heats up. The frog doesn't realize his body is getting dangerously hot. And I didn't realize I was getting dangerously out of shape until it was almost too late. I began to pack on pounds in my late twenties. And I added more in my thirties and forties. Over the span of about 25 years, I had accumulated 75 pounds of unwanted fat. That's a lot of fat but it's just three pounds each year for a quarter of a century.

Then one day I woke up and realized I was obese. I wasn't just a little overweight. I had crossed all the way through 50 pounds of being overweight and had sprawled another 25 pounds into the obese category.

In hindsight, I'm sure I must have realized I was on the wrong track. I made some decisions along the way to slow the train wreck that was about to unfold but I couldn't get switched to the track I wanted to travel. For example, I remained physically active. Perhaps not consistently, but I would train for a half-marathon and complete it, pat myself on the back and go celebrate with another pizza. Or I would ride a century (one hundred mile bike ride) and tell myself I was still reasonably fit. But the hills got harder to climb each year and my growing weight made the exercise less enjoyable. When my cholesterol spiked I made a dietary change and gave up red meat. That seemed to help keep my cholesterol levels under 200 but my triglycerides were still at risk from all the processed flour and sugar I was consuming.

By the time I turned 50 my health condition was in a mess. I was in a very stressful job, I weighed 270 pounds, I hadn't run or biked in more than five years and other than intermittent walking, I wasn't getting any exercise at all. My diet was horrible. Though I was still avoiding red meat, I replaced meat with processed cheese or chicken dishes along with other processed foods composed of sugar or corn syrup, "refined" flour, fats and supplemented with more chemicals than I could pronounce. Something in my life needed to change.

That very year Dad and I made a trip together to Ethiopia. I was leading a team of college students to volunteer for three weeks at a remote school administered by Project Mercy. Dad had agreed to join us to help provide support and to see for himself the holistic program offered by Project Mercy. While we were there, Dad presented an overview to the team on steps for healthy living. I had heard most of this information before but it was a good refresher and I took notes with the intention of implementing Dad's good advice when I got home. As had been the case too many times before, I returned home to the same old lifestyle and same old stresses that quickly overshadowed my good intentions. Despite losing weight in Ethiopia and keeping it off for a few weeks, the next three months saw me pack all the lost weight back on, and add a couple more pounds for good measure.

I was discouraged but not defeated. Despite many failed attempts to regain my health, I made the decision to try once more. And this time I

determined to do whatever was required, to take every step needed, to suc-
cessfully achieve my weight loss goals. This mindset was my first step and
it has become my **First** recommendation—make up your mind that you
can determine your own health. No one else could do this for me. I needed
to have the right positive attitude and the willingness to do whatever was
necessary each day to move toward improved health. *"Believe in yourself!
Have faith in your abilities! Without a humble but reasonable confidence in
your own powers you cannot be successful or happy."*—Norman Vincent Peale

My **Second** goal was to break my addiction to processed carbohydrates,
especially refined sugar and flour. So I began to make changes to my diet,
focusing on replacing foods high in calories with foods high in nutritional
value. And that has become my second recommendation—eat more nutritional whole foods. I cut out the processed sweets, breads and fats, replacing them with natural foods like vegetables, fruits, beans, nuts, seeds and
whole grains. *"The foods with the highest micronutrient per calorie scores are
green vegetables, colorful vegetables, and fresh fruits. For optimal health and to
combat disease, it is necessary to consume enough of these foods that deliver the
highest concentration of nutrients."* —Dr. Joel Fuhrman

The **Third** thing I needed to do was burn more calories. That meant
exercise. I focused on two types of activities, cardiovascular exercise and
strength training. My goal was and is to engage in at least one of these
activities for at least 30 minutes each day, at least six days each week. *"It
[exercise] is the secret to great health. You should exercise hard almost every
day of your life - say six days a week. Exercise is the great key to aging."* —Dr.
Henry Lodge

The **Fourth** change I made was to fully hydrate my body every day. In
some ways, this required the most discipline but I am confident that this
was one of the most important commitments I made. So I strongly recommend that everyone who wants to lose weight drink more water. The exact
amount each person needs will vary based on body size, activity levels and

the season of year but in general, each person should drink at least one ounce of water for every two pounds of total body weight. For me, I started out with more than a gallon of water daily. I think I probably lost a few pounds just running to the men's room more often! But I recorded every ounce I drank and tried to distribute my water consumption evenly throughout the day. *"Water helps to maintain your ideal weight by increasing metabolism and regulating appetite."* —Water Your Body

My *Fifth* suggestion is to record all this in a daily log. Throughout my journey I recorded my daily weight, daily blood pressure, my daily exercise, and everything I put in my mouth. This discipline of journaling creates a form of accountability that makes it more difficult to cheat, especially if you allow someone else to review what you record. So for record-keeping, encouragement and accountability, I recommend each person keep a daily journal. To make this a little more convenient, I got one of the phone apps that calculates calories burned and calories consumed. Since I carry my phone everywhere I go, I always have my food and exercise journal with me and I can track progress through weekly reports. In addition, I can allow significant others to encourage my progress along the way. *"After adjusting for race, gender, and initial weight, greater weight loss was associated with [the] number of food records kept per week."* —Jack Hollis, PhD

My *Sixth* recommendation is to follow the advice of Benjamin Franklin. "Early to bed, early to rise, makes a man healthy, wealthy and wise." I can't say much about wealth or wisdom but I have definitely experienced abundant health as I have followed Mr. Franklin's advice. In the winter months I rose each weekday at 4:30 a.m. And after two hours of moderate to vigorous exercise, I would still have an hour to shower, eat breakfast and make the ten minute drive to work by 7:30 a.m. One of the great side effects of this schedule is that by 8:30 p.m., I was ready for bed and I could sleep soundly through the night. As spring turned into summer, longer daylight made it more challenging to settle down before dark. So I have chosen to sleep in until 5 a.m. but I still make it a point to do cardio or strength training each morning before work. And I still make it a point to try to go to bed by 9 or 9:30 p.m. For me, that kind of faithful discipline can only be assured with an early start to the day.

My **Seventh** piece of advice is to pursue joyful living with someone you care about! I can't emphasize enough the benefits that are associated with association. For me, that primary social connection is with my healthy and beautiful wife, Colleen. Throughout my weight loss journey, she rose early with me, exercised with me, drank water with me, ate buckets of salad with me, and though she didn't need to make changes as much as I did, she too experienced healthy benefits from our renewed commitments. In addition to each other, we had the support of other family members like our children, our parents and extended family. Our friends in our weekly reading group adjusted habits to include fresh fruit at every gathering and when weather permitted, we often met to walk local trails and catch up with each other while exercising! *"Two are better than one because they have a good return for their labor. For if either of them falls, the one will lift up his companion. But woe to the one who falls when there is not another to lift him up."* —Ecclesiastes 4:9-10

Statistics:

I am six feet, four inches tall and I started my weight loss journey at an obese weight of 272 pounds, a BMI of 33 and with 39 percent Body Fat. I was on prescription medication for hypertension with blood pressure measurements consistently above 140/110. I was almost always tired from inadequate rest and inactivity. In addition, I struggled with poor digestion from a horrible diet.

I had determined that I was going to do everything I could to reach a healthy weight and BMI within one year. My initial goals were to lose 50 pounds in the first six months and 25 pounds more in the second half of the year to bring my weight under 200 pounds and my BMI under 25. My subsequent goal was to maintain a weight under 200 pounds into the future. I also set a goal to bring my blood pressure down to a healthy level without medication and get my cholesterol and triglycerides within recommended ranges.

While I am convinced this commitment can be initiated at any time of year, I started with a New Year's resolution. But about the only changes I made on January 1 were that I stopped eating sweets and started recording everything I ate on my *Lose It!* app. (*Lose It!* also offers reports, motivators, badges to mark progress and an online social networking opportunity for people trying to lose weight.) Then, I departed on January 4 for two weeks in Ethiopia. While there I did a lot of walking and I ate a lot of natural whole food including injera (a bread made from whole-grain tef) and wat (stew made from vegetable and lean meats). By the time I returned two weeks later from Ethiopia, I was down about 15 pounds and I lost about five more in the next few days just re-adjusting. This first 20 pounds came off in three weeks with minimal effort on my part. But with that good start to help get me motivated, I decided to get serious about my health goals.

Immediately upon returning home, and while my body was still on Ethiopia time, I started rising each morning at 4:30 to work out for two hours before going to work. (Tip: I used a sunrise alarm clock with 30 minute graduated light to help the body start adjusting before awakening and I woke up feeling ready to get started rather than groggy and averse to light). I started working out pretty easy, doing Wii Fit balance and light aerobic exercises. Then I started doing a little Yoga and walking on the treadmill.

I also started attending a weight-loss program and gained motivation from the accountability of weekly weigh-ins. I supplemented the program by reading everything I could about better health, fitness and weight loss. Some of the best titles I read include:

Secret of the Non-Diet by Dr. Rudy Kachmann

Eat to Live by Dr. Joel Fuhrman

Younger Next Year by Dr. Henry Lodge and Chris Crowley

The Bowflex Body Plan by Dr. Ellington Darden

And what I learned resulted in the following lifestyle changes:

- I now exercise every day (at least six days each week) with heart-pumping, heavy-breathing cardio exercise four days each week and strength training three days each week.

- I eat healthy every day, focusing on getting the most nutritional value for my calorie buck.

- I quit eating C.R.A.P. (Caffeine, Refined Sugar and Flour, Additives, Preservatives)

- I consume about two thirds of my calories from vegetables (half raw, half cooked) and fresh fruit. For my remaining calories, I try to eat beans or legumes daily along with a handful of nuts (preferably raw), and a tablespoon of ground flaxseed.

- I limit animal products to occasional fish, very little poultry, and no beef or pork.

- I place more value on caring relationships in my life.

  - I love those dearest to me and let them know how much I care.

  - I work hard to make those relationships a priority.

  - I involve myself in worthwhile causes, working to make a difference for good.

As I learned more about healthy living, I began applying myself more to nutrition and exercise. By February I was doing strength training with

Bowflex® resistance and free weights three days each week, doubling up with both strength and cardio workouts on Saturdays. As weather permitted, I also started increasing distance and speed in my outdoor walks and gradually began incorporating light jogging. In March, Colleen and I enrolled in a weekly step class at church and purchased an exercise DVD for additional workouts at home (for days when weather made going outside difficult).

In April we registered for a local 10K and completed the course in the rain with smiles on our faces. Then in June I completed my first triathlon with our 21-year-old son. The course included a five-hundred yard swim, a ten mile bike ride and a three mile run. My goals were simple: don't drown, don't fall and don't walk. I certainly didn't threaten the elite athletes but I finished with a smile and enjoyed myself so much I did my second triathlon a week later and my third just three weeks after that.

The Results:

Within six months, my weight had dropped 75 pounds to just under 200 pounds and my BMI was down from obese to normal at about 24. My body fat percentage is under 19 percent. My average blood pressure is about 112/74 with a resting heart rate around 58. I have been off blood pressure medication since my sixth week on this program. My total cholesterol is at 117 with HDL's at 31 and LDL's at 73. My triglycerides are at 66. Through diet and exercise, I have reversed the symptoms of premature aging.

While I am grateful to be able to report these healthy numbers, what is more important to me is that I have abundant energy for activities with my family and abundant joy in my life! I feel better today than I have felt in decades. I am once again experiencing the joys of healthy living! And I am confident that if they follow Dad's recommendations, almost everyone can experience comparable benefits!

CHAPTER THREE

Your Story

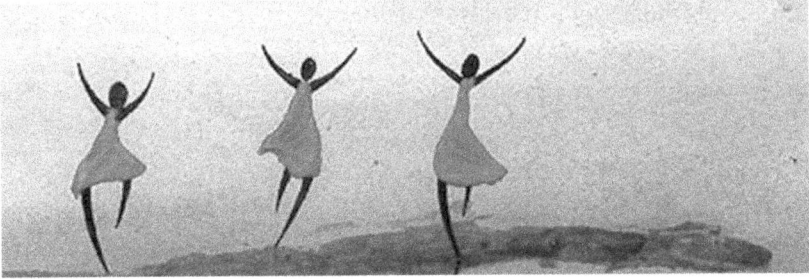

Discover Your Inner Health Power

Your health story is unique. You are the only one who knows it intimately. No one knows how it will evolve in the future. Since you picked this book up, chances are you're looking for ways to improve your health in some way. If so, you've picked up the right book. Your inner health power is greater than you realize. My purpose is to help you discover how to use your inner health power to improve your life and health more than you may think possible.

You may have turned much responsibility for your health over to others in the past, thinking that the "experts" know more than you do about health. That may be true as a generality, but most of the medical world is wrapped up in the overwhelming demands of disease diagnosis and care. The views of many medical specialists are often quite narrowly focused on the disease they are trained to treat. Their views may not be laser-sharp when it comes to your best route to long-term overall health.

The truth is that you have more power to nurture your own good health than anyone else does, even the best of doctors. You are the one with reason to stand up for your own health. You are the only one who can live your life. The person you must rely on for your health is you yourself. The good news is that you have an inner health genius —a helper you may have overlooked until now. Who is this genius? It's your own subconscious mind working in collaboration with your body's incredible cellular wisdom.

Your body has trillions of cells—a number that's hard to imagine, let alone think about managing, but that's just the tip of the management challenge. We now know that each cell has millions of micro-functions going on simultaneously—functions that are essential for the ongoing maintenance and operation of your body. Furthermore, these millions of micro-functions must be coordinated with those of trillions of other cells in your body, or you would simply be a mass of quivering protoplasm instead of an intelligent, purposeful human being.

Could your conscious mind handle this management challenge? Not by itself. It would be snowed under with a fraction of this responsibility. Yet, your subconscious mind, working with your body's natural healing wisdom, handles it all beautifully, without your ever giving it a conscious thought. Your innate natural healing power is indeed magnificent.

Then why do we get into serious health trouble? Why do things go haywire in our bodies? A major reason is that the work of the subconscious mind and the body's natural healing power is complicated by unwise choices we make with the conscious mind. Many actions or habits initiated by the conscious mind interfere with the inner workings of the body so badly that we begin suffering from serious disorders or diseases of one kind or another. Consider the following examples.

Making poor dietary choices can lead to cholesterol plaques clogging up vital arteries in our bodies. This is common and more devastating than most people realize. Arteries supply every cell in the body with oxygen and nutrients essential to life and health. When delivery of these vital nutrients to cells is blocked or even partially blocked, they cannot function as they should. Serious cellular malfunction contributes to disease or degenerative disorders that progressively limit health. Unfortunately, this kind of arterial disease has become the rule instead of the exception in most of the world today.

Smoking tobacco damages the delicate alveolar structure of the lungs over time, all too often leading to chronic lung disease or cancer. It also interferes with microcirculation to cells throughout the body, aggravating many of the same kinds of health problems caused by blockage of arterial lifelines by cholesterol plaques.

Chemical pollution of the body can interfere with vital micro-functions of millions of cells. Other unwise choices can lead to serious compromise of the immune systems so vital to protecting our health. Sedentary lifestyles can eventually lead to multiple kinds of serious health problems. In short, poor conscious choices can severely undermine the work of our unconscious minds and sabotage the natural healing power of our bodies.

Even when we begin suffering major health problems, our healing power is greater than most of us realize. If we give our minds and bodies the kind of support they need, they can correct many serious disorders to a remarkable degree. Our internal healing power is that great. How do we harness this power? Here is a brief outline of the basic steps one can take. We'll go into each step more thoroughly in Part II of this book.

Steps to Take

The *first step* is to choose highly nutritious foods that strengthen and protect health in multiple ways. This includes lots of plant-based foods that boost your immune systems and invigorate the internal functions of your body. Eat these foods abundantly.

The **second step** is to avoid or minimize sabotaging kinds of food and drink that interfere with the inner workings of your body at the cellular level. A corollary to this principle is to avoid inhaling or introducing damaging chemicals to your body. It's hard for your body to work well with microscopic or sub-microscopic debris clogging your inner life-sustaining operations. When these processes are damaged, our operating efficiency suffers, and when this becomes severe, we are subject to serious disorders.

The **third healing step** is to maintain your physical activity and rest patterns in good balance. The key word is balance. Both rest and activity are essential for optimal health. Too much or not enough of either does not help the body.

The **fourth step** to is to practice good hygiene. Most people understand that hand-washing is important for overall hygiene. It's essential in helping to prevent transmission of infections, and it's symbolic of good hygiene. Fewer people realize the importance of good mental hygiene. Yet great spiritual masters through the ages have taught that toxic thoughts are damaging. Modern psychologists agree. Good mental hygiene is vital to overall health.

The **fifth step** is to make sure your connections with yourself and others are positive. Positive relationships with yourself and those around you are essential for long-term good health of both mind and body.

The **final step** important for good long-term healing is the practice of devoting oneself to some quiet time daily. This is not high on the radar screen for many people, but its value for well-being is greater than most people realize.

That's it. These six simple steps provide the tools and the space that your body and mind need to do their healing work. These steps are based on solid science. They are easy to understand, but making such lifestyle changes is easier said than done. The challenge is that our cultural environment today presents many obstacles that must be sidestepped to put these simple steps into practice.

One of the toughest challenges we face in our quest for healthy living is mental. If your mind tells you that the path to healthy living is too difficult, it will be. On the other hand, if you decide, "I can do this," you can find the inner resources to achieve the healthy lifestyle you truly want. We will go into each step more thoroughly later in the book

Summary of Six Simple Steps to Healthy Living

I'll close this chapter with a concise summary of the six simple steps to healthy living. Write them down. Tape them on your refrigerator, your bathroom mirror, the cover of your health journal, or on all three places. This will help you absorb them deeply into your mind. Join me in learning how to make these steps a vital part of your life. Your story will become what you want it to be.

1. Avoid health-sabotaging foods, drinks and substances.

2. Eat highly nutritious foods frequently and abundantly.

3. Keep physical activity and rest in good balance.

4. Practice good hygiene of body, mind and soul.

5. Nourish good connections with oneself and others.

6. Maintain a daily practice of quality quiet time.

The Power of Lifestyle

(Each chapter from chapter four to fifteen will have one or two introductory paragraphs in italics to dramatize the theme of the chapter. A fictional character named Adam represents all humans in the ways they could be impacted by the chapter's theme.)

Eat Wholesome Foods Abundantly

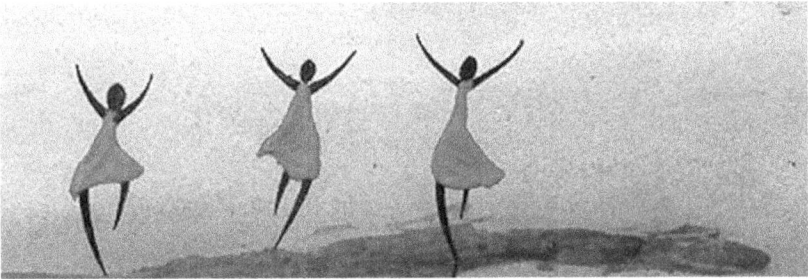

Food is the foundation of good health. Paradoxically, it can also be danger-ously treacherous. Wholesome plant-based foods support Adam better than any other foods. Veggies and fruits are among the best anti-aging foods known. In addition to strongly promoting good health, they defend Adam from hordes of free radicals and other deceptive attackers, including other foods that may be very tasty. Adam often favors the latter, not understanding they are saboteurs, and not realizing that veggies and fruits are his strong allies and stout defend-ers if given half a chance.

Food A Powerful Factor in Health

The power of lifestyle begins at the table. Food is one of our most powerful determinants of health. Wholesome foods nurture good health in many marvelous ways. Yet, poor food choices can undermine health badly. Clearly, it's vital to know which foods support good health as well as which ones sabotage health. It's best to avoid or minimize the saboteurs. We'll learn more about them in the next chapter.

First we'll look at foods that are good for health. Many of them are ones that most people enjoy, such as fruits like apples, bananas, peaches and strawberries. These foods are full of vitamins and other nutrients that help build good health. Most fruits and vegetables are good for our health. As a general rule, if a food is colorful, it is likely to have abundant vitamins, antioxidants, and other nutrients that are good for us. A nutritional truism states that the more colorful one's plate of food is, the healthier it's likely to be.

Some people avoid eating many or most vegetables, saying they don't like them. While that may be true, most of us can re-train our tastes if we are motivated to do so. Many people acquire tastes for foods as they mature that they did not like when they were younger. When I was a kid, I didn't care for foods like okra, kale, collard greens, and mushrooms, but today they are among my favorite foods. Food tastes are culturally determined for the most part, and we can re-educate our taste buds!

Value of Plant-Based Foods

There are several reasons why fruits and vegetables are so good for us. Aside from the fact that they are loaded with vitamins and other vital nutrients, plants are the only forms of life that have the ability to convert the sun's energy into food energy. No other living things can do this. Because they convert the sun's energy into food energy, plants provide us with the cleanest food energy available on planet Earth. They are the most potent anti-aging foods known.

Animals get their energy from plants. This is true even of animals that are strictly meat-eaters, because they eat animals that are plant-eaters. All food energy ultimately comes through plants that convert the sun's photons into food by photosynthesis. Plant-based foods give us clean primary energy, whereas food energy that comes from animal sources is always second or third-hand energy. Primary sources are usually the best.

In addition to the fact that plants provide us with our best sources of energy, most of them are low in calories. A person can eat platefuls of such food without gaining excess weight. Although they are low in calories, they are more filling than most other foods because they have a lot of bulk. The result is that one feels full and satisfied after eating a meal of this remarkable food, and yet one's calorie intake remains reasonable.

One reason that whole plant-based foods are filling even though they are low in calories is that they contain more water than most other foods. Many fruits and vegetables are 80 to 90 percent water by weight. This water is good for us in many ways. Yet, it carries no calories whatsoever. Our own bodies are about 60 percent water, so the water we get in the plant-based foods we eat is something that our bodies crave. It's a real boost to health.

Another reason that plant food is bulkier than animal-based food is that plants are full of fiber. Fiber is another ingredient that is great for health, but carries no calories. Fiber is more valuable for health than we knew 50 years ago. It comes in both soluble and insoluble forms in the plant-based foods we eat, and both forms are good for us. Insoluble fiber adds bulk to our bowel contents, making them easier to move through the intestinal tract.

Soluble fiber dissolves in water, forming a gel that absorbs cholesterol and carries it out of the body, making it a valuable help in controlling cholesterol. It also softens bowel contents and lowers the risk of constipation.

Whole grains, nuts and beans are rich in fiber as well as many other nutrients. Nuts are high in calories because of their high fat content and should be eaten in moderation. Avocados and olives are other high-fat foods, being among the few plant-based foods that are high in fat. The fats involved provide omega-3 and omega-6 fats that are essential for human health. Although they are sources of good fat, these foods are high in calories, so it's wise to eat them in limited quantities

Most plant-based foods have an alkaline effect in the body after being digested, providing another significant benefit from eating lots of fruits and vegetables. Our blood is slightly alkaline, having a pH of 7.4 that the body must preserve to remain healthy. If this pH becomes even slightly acidic, it can be fatal. Since plant-based foods have a natural alkaline impact on the body, they are easy for the body to metabolize and are good for health.

Summary

To summarize, wholesome plant-based foods are great for health. A vital source of energy, they provide abundant vitamins, antioxidants and fiber in packages that are tasty but usually low in calories. They help the body maintain a desirable pH level, assist in the natural control of desirable cholesterol levels, and help preserve youthful vitality. This is not an exhaustive review of their benefits, but it's enough to highlight the fact that they are valuable foods, essential for the goal of achieving lifelong well-being!

CHAPTER FIVE

Minimize Sabotaging Foods!

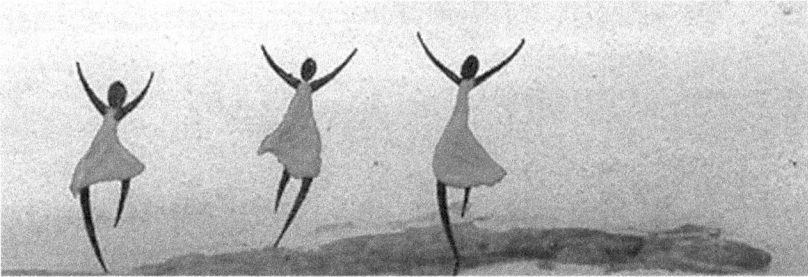

Junk foods and other rogue elements assault Adam in various ways, especially by attacking his arteries. Tobacco smoke, sugar, high fructose corn syrup, assorted high-fat foods, and other agents are among those assailing these vital lifelines. Why doesn't Adam evade these attacks? He doesn't realize he's under attack. Despite having diseased arteries, he looks perfectly healthy outwardly. If the inner damage from this warfare was visible, he would soon spurn the saboteurs.

The Hidden Health Problem

What are "sabotaging foods," and why are they a concern? When I speak or write of, "sabotaging foods," I mean foods that seriously undermine health. However, health is a broad subject and the ways that food undermines it are a bit fuzzy, so it's hard to see this problem clearly. Because of this, it's helpful to narrow the problem down more specifically to understand what is really at stake.

Atherosclerosis is a hidden health problem for many people, but it is a good proxy for general health for several reasons. One of the reasons is that it is a serious contributing factor to many major disorders, including most heart disease, strokes, kidney failure, blindness, peripheral arterial disease, and impotence among men. Another reason is that it is widespread in our adult population, more so than most people realize. Finally, while we haven't fully unraveled all the complex causes of atherosclerosis, we have a fair understanding of them today.

Atherosclerosis is a hidden problem for most people because it's not visible and because it does not cause any symptoms for decades as it develops. Symptoms may appear when the disease is far advanced, but the first symptoms can be catastrophic. A fatal stroke or heart attack may be the first outward sign of disease. Seeing a picture of a diseased artery makes the severity of this problem very clear. Look at this picture carefully. Would you want this artery as a major lifeline in your body?

Atherosclerotic Aorta

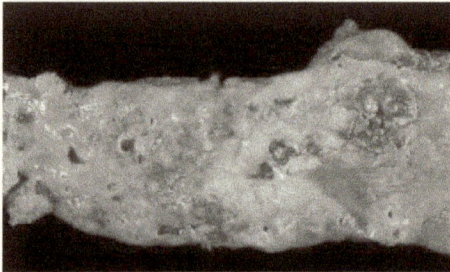

Today we know that atherosclerosis begins in the early teens and is pervasive among most Americans by their mid-thirties. How do we know? A major autopsy study of 2876 black and white men, women and youth between the ages of 15 to 34 was reported in the *Journal of the American Medical Association* in 1999. All subjects had fatty streaking evident in some of their arteries at all ages. Over half of them had raised atherosclerotic plaques occurring by their thirties.

The sobering thing about this study is that the subjects were not known in advance to have arterial disease. Autopsies were done because they had died from some external form of violence. Yet evidence of early atherosclerosis was present in all 15-year-olds, and it had progressed to more serious disease in a majority of all subjects by their thirties. What this means is that most Americans have significant arterial disease even if they don't know about it. It's a hidden health problem.[1]

What Causes Atherosclerosis?

There's no single cause of atherosclerosis. It is the result of the interplay of multiple factors. While science still hasn't put the total picture together of how this disease is caused, after decades of intensive research, we have a better understanding of its multiple causes. The National Heart, Lung and Blood Institute summarizes this by stating that at least four major factors are involved in causing widespread damage to arteries. Over time, plaque builds up at many of these sites, producing atherosclerotic disease.[2]

Four major factors involved in causing this damage over time include: (1) smoking; (2) high blood pressure; (3) high levels of LDL cholesterol and certain other fats; and (4) high levels of blood sugar due to insulin resistance. Not all these factors are necessary to cause atherosclerosis, but the more of them that are involved, the higher the risk becomes. We'll look at the first two factors briefly, and then we'll spend a bit more time on the last two, which are the main focus of this chapter.

Tobacco smoke has thousands of chemicals in it, including the nicotine that makes it so addictive. They cause serious injury to the lungs, but many

---

1. Strong, J.P., et al. "Prevalence and Extent of Atherosclerosis in Adolescents and Young Adults." *Journal of the American Medical Association*, February 24, 1999—Vol. 281, No. 8, p.735.

2. http://www.nhlbi.nih.gov/health/health-topics/topics/atherosclerosis/causes.html

of these chemicals also get into the blood stream of smokers where they cause inflammatory damage to the inner lining of the arteries. Such damage sets the arteries up for the subsequent development of atherosclerosis.

High blood pressure causes microscopic breaks in the endothelium of arteries at stress points. Inflammatory changes occur around these microscopic breaks, and atherosclerosis often develops at such stress points. Smoking in combination with high blood pressure nearly doubles the risk of severe atherosclerosis and its many complications.

High cholesterol and high blood sugar levels also increase the risk of atherosclerosis, though in different ways. In spite of decades of research, science still has some questions as to precisely how these factors cause damage, but it's clear that they are involved. Because of sometimes conflicting research reports, there has been confusion about these risk factors.

There is even more confusion about the choices of foods one should eat or not eat to avoid these risks. Many kinds of health diets have been proposed. Some of these are based on mistaken information or are pushed by commercial interests, or both. With all the controversy, it's no wonder that the public is confused about this.

Still, there is solid scientific information about sugar and cholesterol that is worth noting and remembering. I will discuss this briefly and then give you my view of what this means in terms of making healthy food choices. First, let's look at what we know about cholesterol and sugar and their impact on health.

Cholesterol and Sugar

Cholesterol is a waxy, fat-like substance that is normally part of every cell in the body. Our bodies also use cholesterol to make a variety of hormones and other essential substances. The body makes the cholesterol it needs, but some of the foods we eat also affect cholesterol levels. Cholesterol is carried through the blood stream as either low-density (LDL) or high density (HDL) lipoprotein packets. (Lipoproteins are molecules that combine fat and protein.)

There are several kinds of LDL cholesterol. One kind in particular is involved with causing inflammation in arterial walls at sites where there are microscopic breaks in its lining. Eventually, this complex inflammatory process leads to the formation of atheromas that threaten normal blood flow. Most other cholesterol fractions seem to be innocent, which may explain why much cholesterol research has produced confusing and controversial results. However, it's clear that LDL cholesterol is involved in atheroma formation.

Refined sugar is also a problem. Sugar is found naturally in many fruits and vegetables. The problem is that since humans learned to extract sucrose from sugar cane, we consume more than our bodies were designed to use. The average person today eats far more sugar than was true in 1700 (four pounds/year in 1700 vs 150 pounds/year in 2010.) It's this excess sugar intake that causes health problems. The nutritional content of sugar cane is lost in the refining process. Sugar is empty of all value except calories. In 1997 the World Health Organization said sugar had "zero nutritional value."

High Fructose Corn Syrup (HFCS) is in a similar situation. These two sweeteners are consumed more heavily than most people realize. In the USA, the average person consumes over 20 teaspoons daily without being aware of it, because most sugar and HFCS is hidden in soft drinks and a host of other processed foods. Both sucrose (table sugar) and HFCS consist of glucose and fructose in slightly different concentrations. (For convenience sake, I'll use the word sugar to cover both sucrose and HFCS from now on, unless otherwise specified.)

High blood sugar levels cause insulin resistance to develop, increase the production of free radicals, stimulate conversion of excess sugar to fatty triglycerides, and drive the production of advanced glycation end-products

(AGEs). What this means is that excess sugar intake increases the risk of atherosclerosis in multiple ways. Each of these ways deserves a separate chapter to explain fully, but the bottom line for all of them is that excess sugar is a serious hazard to long-term health.

Today we know that prediabetes, a condition due to excess sugar intake, can precede the development of type 2 diabetes for many years. People with prediabetes have no tell-tale symptoms, but they carry a risk of cardiovascular disease similar to people with full-blown type 2 diabetes. The American Heart Association has become so concerned about the evidence linking high sugar intake to these problems that it advises limiting sugar intake to nine teaspoons a day or less for men, and six teaspoons a day or less for women.

What Foods Pose Serious Threats to Health?

Past research indicated that eating foods high in saturated fats increase LDL levels the most, and that saturated fat intake should be minimized as much as possible. More recently, trans fats have been found to pose a greater threat to health than saturated fat, and so foods with trans fats have been added to the list of foods to be minimized. (Most trans fats consist of polyunsaturated vegetable oils, such as corn oil, with hydrogen added to unsaturated fat molecules.)

The foods that are highest in saturated fats are basically meat and dairy products. Partially hydrogenated vegetable oils, sometimes called trans fats, are found in a great variety of processed foods because they are so commercially useful. Examples of such foods include cakes, pies, cookies, candies, chips, deep-fried foods, and many canned and bottled food products. Since labeling of trans fat on food labels became required by law, the use of trans fat has dropped, but it's still used enough to make reading of labels a good idea. (The law only requires labeling of trans fat if there is over 1/2 gram per food serving, so some foods still have trans fat even though the labeling doesn't show this. In November 2013, the Food and Drug Administration announced plans to phase all added trans fats out of all processed foods in the future because they are so health-damaging.)

To complicate matters, high sugar intake raises triglyceride and LDL levels in a complex series of steps. To summarize this process in lay terms, the liver essentially turns into a fat factory when driven by high sugar intake. Much of this fat is stored in fat cells around the body, but some becomes involved in complex cholesterol processes that damage the arteries. This is over-simplification, but it's on target. Consuming too much sugar clearly leads to multiple health hazards.[3]

The USA and the entire world has experienced an obesity epidemic in the last 40 years never seen before. Two thirds of all Americans are overweight, and half of these overweight people are obese. It is more than a problem of appearances, for the obesity epidemic is fueling many other serious health problems today. Many factors are involved, but excess sugar consumption contributes to the problem.

Fructose intake has escalated sharply since HFCS was adopted for commercial sweetening purposes in 1970. We know that the body cannot use all this excess fructose. The liver converts most of this into triglycerides (fat) that is stored in fat cells throughout the body. The linkage between excess fructose consumption and the development of obesity is strong!

Type 2 diabetes is another health problem that has exploded in epidemic proportions over the past 40 years. Excess sugar consumption is a significant factor in this disease. It is intertwined with the obesity epidemic in that obese people are more likely to become diabetic than non-obese people. The challenge of treating millions of people with these health issues and their complications strains the health budgets of countries around the world.

The final sugar-related problem is premature aging. Excess glucose and

---

3. http://circ.ahajournals.org/content/123/20/2292.long

fructose bind with protein in the body in a process called glycation. This protein has reduced elasticity and is functionally impaired. The net effect is premature aging of tissues and organs throughout the body. Limiting sugar intake may be one of the best ways to maintain youthful vitality longer!

Another highly processed food is refined white flour. The bran and much of the wheat germ is stripped away in the refining process, and the end product has less nutritional value than its whole wheat counterpart. Whole wheat has more protein, five times as much fiber, and twice as much calcium as refined flour.

Refined white flour is sometimes called "enriched" because a few of the vitamins lost in processing are added back at the end. Even so, "enriched refined flour" is a nutritional ghost. Virtually all the bran and fiber, and most of the vitamins and antioxidants found in the original whole grain are gone. Unfortunately, for those who are gluten-sensitive, refined white flour has a high gluten content, providing another good reason to avoid white flour. Gluten-sensitive people need to look for other flours that are specifically gluten-free.

Conclusion

To conclude, scientific research has given us more nutritional information than we had 50 years ago, but we still have some nutritional enigmas. Realizing that we'll have better information in the future, my recommendations are based on what we know today. My evaluation is based on the review of scientific literature on food and health that I've done through the years. I test each of my food recommendations by applying what I learn in my own life. My body is my laboratory.

Simply to let you know the facts, the results are good up to this point in my life. My body is in good shape at age 77. I take no medications. My blood pressure is consistently around 110/70. My blood chemistries are all in excellent balance. I'm a hearty eater, but my BMI stays close to 21 with no need to ever count calories. I enjoy an active life, play tennis two or three times a week, and take pleasure in my daily walks and evening gardening. I also love the volunteer teaching and the mountain hiking I do at Africa University each year. To sum it up, I find abundant joy in life.

Following are my personal rules regarding foods that undermine health:

1. Minimize foods that are high in saturated and/or trans fats. These foods include fatty meats and highly processed meats like sausage and most cold cuts. It also includes most dairy products except for those labeled non-fat.

2. Minimize sugars of all kinds.

3. Minimize other refined carbs. This includes white flour in particular, and all the foods made with it.

These rules are simple in concept and easy to remember. They are not as easy to apply. I know, because I struggled with this issue myself over the years. Unfortunately, many of our most popular foods fall into this category, and I loved most of them as a young person. It took me years to wean myself off of them.

As a teenager, I loved *Three Musketeers* candy bars. They only cost a nickel then, and I had one every day on the way home from school. When I went to college, I had to earn my way with low-paying college jobs (35 cents an hour), and I couldn't afford to keep up my candy habit. I never returned to my love affair with the *Three Musketeers*, but that didn't stop my liking for sweets. I worked in our college cafeteria, and I topped off every meal with a great piece of pie or cake.

Later, as I reviewed more nutritionally-related research articles, my motivation to eat became more health-oriented. Over the years, I gradually dropped cake, pie, cookies, ice cream and various pastries from my daily diet.

My suggestion for anyone struggling with cutting down on any of these foods is to do so gradually, but it can be done more quickly than I did. Ultimately, the degree to which you minimize these foods is up to you. The degree of benefit you will reap is likely to be related to the degree of control you have over them.

Today, I avoid or minimize all such foods. Do I miss any of them? My honest answer is "No." Looking back, I have no regrets at all. I enjoy my healthy breakfasts, lunches and suppers so much that I don't miss the old meats and sweets at all. Our desserts today almost always consist of fresh fruit.

Dr. Lee Coleman answered a similar question several years ago after he lost 170 pounds by engaging in a healthy exercise and eating program. When asked if he didn't miss his old favorites, he said, "I retrained my mind to love the healthy foods so much that I lost interest in the unhealthy items." He added this qualification: "If a person doesn't change their mindset towards healthy eating, the new lifestyle may be difficult to maintain."[4]

I agree with him completely. (If you wish to read more about Dr. Coleman's story, check reference #4.)

---

4. http://www.everydayhealth.com/columns/weight-loss-success-stories/170-pounds-lost-dr-lee-coleman-jr-walks-the-weight-off-and-sets-an-example/

CHAPTER SIX

Foods with a Question Mark

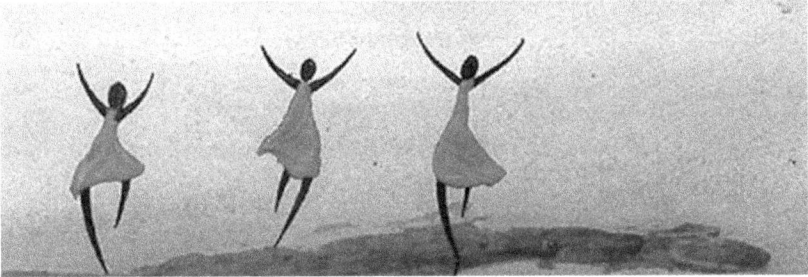

Processed foods are foods that have undergone manmade manipulation to some degree. They pose health risks roughly in proportion to the degree they are processed. The more highly processed they are, the likelier they are to pose significant risks to health. Arteries and the vital organs dependent on them aren't the only ones at risk. The gut and the immune system are also prime targets of trouble-prone processed foods. Other systems are also vulnerable.

Most people are vaguely aware that processed foods may not be ideal, but have little concept of how damaging they can be. Many also don't realize how much processed foods have taken over our daily diet. Some processed foods are now adulterated with "fake" foods that are sold and eaten by unsuspecting customers. This has become such a concern that the "Food Fraud Database" is now published by the official US Pharmacopeial Convention. It's clearly a good idea to learn about foods with a question mark!

Potentially Problematic Foods

A broad range of foods exists between those that clearly enhance health and those that undermine health. In this chapter, we'll look at the in-between foods that carry a question mark concerning their value.

Meat is an example of food that has health benefits, but carries baggage that can undercut health. Meat is a good source of protein, providing all the essential amino acids that humans require. Meat is also a good source of iron needed to make hemoglobin for red blood cells to absorb oxygen for use by cells in every part of the body. So why does meat fall into the category of foods with a question mark? There are several reasons.

All meat has some saturated fat embedded in it, but some meats have much more saturated fat than others. Highly processed meats like sausage, bacon, deli meats, and ground beef have more saturated fat than most other meat, having up to 80 percent of their calories in fat. This makes them very high-calorie foods that increase LDL cholesterol risk. Limiting intake of meat, particularly the kinds of meat that are so high in saturated fat, simply makes good sense. This is true from another standpoint also.

Most meat and dairy products have an acid effect on the body's acid-base balance, which the body must neutralize to safeguard health. The body does this is by leaching calcium from bones, the major reservoir for calcium in the body. Since dissolved calcium is alkaline, it helps keep the blood pH in a safe range, but the dissolved calcium is subsequently filtered through the kidneys and lost in the urine. This acid-base balancing act safeguards life, but does so at a cost to the body that we'll discuss a bit more in a moment.

People eat more meat today than they did a hundred years ago. Food surveys show that many Americans eat more than double the daily recommended amount of protein. Most of the extra protein is in the form of meat. Cutting down on meat helps reduce excess protein intake as well as decrease the hazards posed by saturated fat. Red meat is also linked to increased risk of several kinds of cancer. Many health organizations now advise limiting red meat to no more than two servings a week.

Milk and dairy products are also foods with a question mark. Many dairy products are high in saturated fat, posing health problems similar to those of meat, but even non-fat dairy products are a concern. They are good sources of calcium, but this calcium is not absorbed by the human body as well as calcium from vegetable sources. Acid-base balancing efforts by the body may result in a net loss of calcium from the body in spite of high dairy consumption. This may explain the paradox that countries like the USA and the Scandinavian countries have high rates of osteoporosis and related fractures despite high dairy intake.

Dr. Amy Lanou, on the faculty at the University of North Carolina, discusses this in her book, *Building Bone Vitality*. Her review of over 1200 research studies found that in 72 percent of them, milk, dairy foods and supplemental calcium did not help prevent bone fractures. Humans are the only species that drink milk after infancy. Some of our largest animals, like cattle, buffaloes and elephants, eat only plants, and yet they have the strongest bones in the world. Many people do not realize that foods like broccoli and green leafy vegetables are good sources of calcium, along with many other plant-based foods. Dr. Lanou advises minimizing meat and dairy products, and eating at least two servings of veggies and fruit with every meal as the best way to build bone strength.[5]

There are other health concerns connected with dairy products. Cow's milk is linked to more early childhood problems with allergic and digestive difficulties than is true for breast-fed infants. Casein, one of the main proteins in cow's milk, is linked to increased cancer risks. In view of all the accumulated evidence, I now avoid dairy products.

Other Processed Foods

A tremendous range of processed foods are sold in grocery stores today.

---

5. Amy Joy Lanou, Ph.D., *Building Bone Vitality*, (New York: McGraw Hill, 2009).

It's impractical to go over all of them individually, but except for the fresh produce, most other food items in the store have been processed to some degree. In her book, *What to Eat*, Dr. Marion Nestle makes a useful distinction between lightly processed foods and heavily processed foods. Lightly processed foods are ones like canned or frozen vegetables and fruits that are easily recognized. When you can't tell what the food or original food source is without reading the label, it's probably heavily processed.

Dr. Nestle suggests that the nutritional change in lightly processed foods is so small that they can be eaten as an alternative to fresh produce. Heavily processed foods, however, are changed in significant ways by loss of nutritional value or by additives that add calories (like sugar and fat,) or that distort the value of the original food in other ways. From the standpoint of good nutrition, it's wise to avoid heavily processed foods, or at least minimize them as much as possible.

A number of processed foods are adulterated in various ways today. This has become a growing concern, great enough that the U.S. Pharmacopeial Convention developed a Food Fraud Database that includes more than 1300 entries of food adulteration of some kind. The USP first published the Food Fraud Database in 2012. The amount of damage caused by food fraud is not known, but eating food that has been fraudulently manipulated is certainly not desirable.[6]

Genetically modified foods (GMOs) are manipulated at a deep level, with genes being manipulated in cellular DNA. It's claimed by the biotech companies doing this type of work that no damage is done by such manipulation, but the truth is that nobody knows what the long-term effects will be. The impact of GMO foods on humans and other biological organisms simply hasn't been independently tested over a long enough time period to have any scientific certainty about their value. The reluctance of the biotech companies to allow independent testing is unsettling, as is the willingness

---

6. http://www.foodfraud.org/

of the FDA to forego such testing. In the meantime, eating GMO foods that are genetically adulterated is legally permitted, even though this does not seem wise from a biological perspective.

Vegetable Oil, Fish Oil and Salt

Vegetable oils are processed foods. Some may be better for health than animal-based fats, but there are problems connected with them. Partially hydrogenated vegetable oils are a major concern. This is worth re-emphasizing because trans fats are worse than saturated fat as a risk factor for cardiovascular disease. Identification of trans fats on food labels has led to their reduced use in many commercial foods, but a regulatory loophole permits unlabeled use in food that has less than half a gram per serving. Because of this it's best to avoid any food that lists partially hydrogenated oil as an ingredient. Some foods do not require labeling at all. Many deep-fried foods are cooked in partially hydrogenated oil, so it's best to avoid them as much as possible.

Another concern is that many vegetable oils are unbalanced in their omega-6 to omega-3 ratios. Both of these are essential fats, but we get much more omega-6 fat than omega-3 fat in most of our food. The ideal ratio for omega-6 to omega-3 should be less than 4:1, but many oils and fats in our diets have ratios of 15:1 or even higher. The reason for concern is that high omega-6 intake can trigger inflammatory disease processes in many people. Sources of desirable omega-3 fat include walnuts, flax seeds, and oily fish such as salmon, if caught in the wild. Farm-raised fish do not have this advantage.

Fish oil capsules are taken by many people, but research shows them to be of questionable benefit. Eating oily fish once or twice a week is preferable to taking fish oil capsules. Fish oil capsules are a type of extract, and extracts are rarely as beneficial as the whole food source from which they are taken.

Salt is a common food additive that is heavily used in many commercial foods. It adds an appealing taste to many foods, so it's added to everything from chips and French fries to canned soups. The problem with this from a health point of view is that salt is a major risk factor for high blood pressure and cardiovascular disease. In a report by Harvard researchers at the 2013 American Heart Association meetings, 75 percent of people from all around the world were found to consume nearly twice as much salt as recommended by the World Health Organization (WHO).

According to the Harvard researchers, salt contributed to 2.3 million heart-related deaths around the world in 2010. One in ten deaths in the USA was linked to excess salt intake. Data from the Global Burden of Diseases Study showed that salt consumption was dangerously high in over 180 countries. Only six of 187 countries met the WHO recommended limits on salt intake. Most of us consume too much salt. The best ways to avoid excessive salt are to keep intake of commercial foods to a minimum and to use salt very lightly at home. [7]

Beverages

Most beverages other than water are processed to some degree. Even water is processed when it is bottled or treated chemically but it's the best all-around beverage for us. As noted earlier, our bodies are about 60 percent water, so water is essential for the body. Most other beverages carry some kind of baggage in addition to water, presenting an extra workload for the body since it must unload the extra baggage in order to use the water it truly needs.

Aside from the added workload for the body, the baggage in many beverages is detrimental to health. Most regular sodas have a higher sugar content than most people realize. I discussed sugar problems in the last

7. http://www.huffingtonpost.com/2013/03/21/salt-health-deaths-consump-tion-sodium-heart_n_2916888.html

chapter, but will simply note here that soft drinks are a major source of excess sugar for many people. Artificial sweeteners are substituted for sugar in many beverages labeled as diet drinks. There are at least two concerns about these beverages.

The first is that many artificial sweeteners are of questionable value, and some of them may be detrimental to health. Stevia is an extract from a plant that is naturally sweet, so it may be better than most substitutes. Still, it's an extract that is not useful to the body. The liver must detoxify the natural chemicals in stevia, and then the kidneys eliminate them from the body through urine. They are unnecessary baggage!

Another concern about diet drinks is that they are not effective in helping with weight loss, which is their main purpose. Some research suggests that the sweet taste of diet drinks actually stimulates a greater craving for sweetness. Most people who drink them end up taking in more excess calories from other sources than they avoid in their diet drinks.

Caffeine is another substance that is found in many beverages, most notably coffee and tea. It is also added to some soft drinks and "power" or "energy" drinks. Caffeine has been controversial, and extensive research has been carried out on its health effects. The evidence from all the research is conflicting. There are both good and bad effects from caffeine. The scientific consensus is that, in small amounts, the benefits of caffeine seem to outweigh its undesirable effects. Still, anyone who is sensitive to caffeine should avoid it, and everyone should avoid excessive caffeine. How much is excessive? The jury is still out on this question, but four average cups of coffee in 24 hours is often suggested as a wise upper limit.

The tricky thing about this is that caffeine can also be consumed from other sources, and more may be taken in than realized. The best advice I can give is to read ingredient lists on labels carefully, and avoid consuming too much food or drink with high caffeine levels. I'm caffeine-sensitive, so my personal practice is to avoid all caffeinated food and drinks.

Alcoholic beverages are another controversial topic. As with caffeine, extensive research has been done on the health impact of alcohol. The scientific consensus today is that in small amounts, alcoholic beverages benefit cardiovascular health, but damaging effects increase as alcoholic intake increases. As with caffeine, the tricky thing is defining a safe limit. Most health authorities now recommend limiting alcoholic beverage to not more than one drink daily for women and not more than two drinks daily for men. (One drink can be one can of beer, one five-ounce glass of wine, or a one-ounce serving of hard liquor.) While acknowledging this consensus, my view about safe alcoholic consumption is that less is better.

I recommend lower limits for the following reason. Alcohol is addicting, and the health consequences of excessive alcoholic intake are so devastating that a wide margin of safety is best. One or two drinks a day may be safe if strictly limited to that amount, but even that may start a person down the slippery path of addiction. In my years of practice, I saw social drinking escalate into addiction too often. Because of this "slippery slope" problem, I advise limiting alcoholic beverage to less than one drink a day. This allows an occasional social drink, but avoids consuming alcohol as a daily habit.

Summary

There are concerns about the health impact of many modern processed foods. This review of problematic foods is not exhaustive, but it's enough to help you be aware of the magnitude of the problem. It's clear that making wise food choices is important for health. In the next chapter, we'll look at making good choices in planning and preparing meals.

CHAPTER SEVEN

Create Healthy Meals

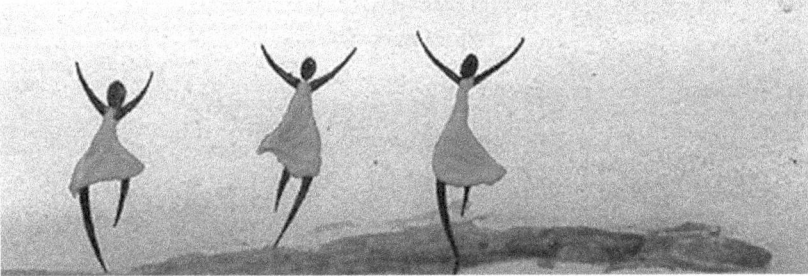

Adam, like most people, falls into a variety of pitfalls and traps in the process of trying to adopt healthier ways of eating. These pitfalls and traps range from skipping meals to skipping healthy food choices to the challenges of eating tempting desserts and eating out. This chapter brings up many of these pitfalls, discusses why each is an issue, and shows ways of dealing with them. We'll also look at the subject of vitamins. At the end of the chapter, Randall, who authored chapter two about his weight struggles, provides practical tips about creating healthy meals that are both nutritious and delicious.

Nutritious Breakfasts

Our meals are based on one bedrock principle: Eat simple wholesome food. First, let's look at meal frequency. Although various approaches are suggested in different books on health, the traditional standard of three wholesome meals a day is supportive of good long-term health.

Some people skip breakfast because they want to lose weight, but careful studies show that skipping breakfast is bad strategy. It simply doesn't work. Those who skip breakfast usually eat excess calories later, especially in the evening or at night, with the result that they gain weight. Skipping breakfast does not help people lose weight.

Others skip breakfast because they don't have time to fix it. This is an excuse that masks the low priority they give breakfast. From a health standpoint, breakfast has high priority for many reasons. Common sense says that the body needs good fuel after being without it all night. Careful studies show that without breakfast, body and mind simply do not function as well as they do with it.[8]

Although missed calories can be made up later in the day, it is difficult to make up for the missed fiber and nutrients that a good breakfast provides. For the sake of one's health, it is wise to take time for a good breakfast.

What constitutes a good breakfast? Good breakfasts offer high nutritional value, good fiber content, and modest calorie intake—a formula that excludes many highly processed foods. The foods that fulfill these criteria best are plant-based foods. Our usual breakfast illustrates this nicely.

We enjoy hot, steel-cut oatmeal, cooked with raisins and topped with sliced banana, strawberries, blueberries, and walnut pieces. Ground cinnamon sprinkled on all this adds a nice taste. I have almond milk on my cereal as a rule, and a side dish of three or four large stewed prunes. I finish breakfast with a cup of hot herbal tea and a slice of whole-wheat toast with organic strawberry jam.

I love this breakfast and look forward to it every morning. Every spoonful provides a variety of tastes, including the tart sweetness of strawberry slices, the mellow soft banana taste, the burst of flavor from an exploding blueberry, and the crunchiness of a piece of walnut, all melded in with the satisfying heartiness of cooked, steel-cut oats. The distinctive taste of ground cinnamon tops it all off. It's great!

A variation of this breakfast is to add amaranth to the steel-cut oats. I

---

8. http://www.kidsource.com/kidsource/content3/ific/ific.breakfast.k12.3.html

add an eighth-cup of amaranth grain to one-half cup of steel-cut oats and stir this in a pan with two cups of water. After bringing it to a boil, I let this mixture simmer for fifteen minutes. This oat-amaranth porridge is a bit chewy with a nutty taste. The amaranth turns a nutritious cereal into a super-nutritious food.

The Amaranth Story

The story of amaranth is fascinating. Amaranth was prized by the Aztecs as the Food of the Gods. It was prepared in religious rituals that involved human sacrifice, horrifying Spanish conquistadores so much that they outlawed its cultivation in all Spanish colonies. Amaranth survived as a wild weed, but its secret use as a food crop was kept alive in a few mountainous villages.

Amaranth truly is a super-food. Emerging from the past, it's now called the food of the future. Analysis proves that in addition to other nutrients, amaranth seed is very high in protein, calcium and iron. This protein is rich in lysine, an essential amino acid rare among plant proteins.

The high lysine content in amaranth sets it apart from other grains. Food scientists regard the protein content of amaranth to be of high "biological value." Amaranth is also high in calcium with 298 milligrams per cup of raw grain compared to 52 milligrams in one cup of raw white rice.[9] In addition to making a good hot cereal, amaranth seed can be added to soups, sprinkled on salads, and even popped like miniature popcorn.

Quinoa is a grain from the same family of plants as amaranth. Both are nutritious. Quinoa is richer in vitamins, while amaranth is higher in some minerals. Quinoa has a slightly bitter taste after cooking that can be avoided by carefully rinsing the grain before cooking. Most quinoa suppliers now do

9. http://glutenfreecooking.about.com/od/nutritionmealplanning/a/amaranth.htm

this before it is sold. We sometimes substitute quinoa for brown rice in our evening meal. It can also be mixed in when cooking a variety of hot cereals.

Cold cereals provide a convenient alternative to hot cereals, but buyers must beware—many cold cereals are high in sugar. Shredded wheat is a good example of a sugarless whole grain cereal that is low in calories. Occasionally we substitute this for hot oatmeal, adding the same kinds of fruit toppings we use with hot cereal.

What about eggs, the mainstay of many breakfasts? Eggs are high in cholesterol and have no fiber. Yet, they do have nutritional value and can be part of a good breakfast if combined with nutritious high-fiber foods such as beans and tomatoes, European-style.

Bacon and all types of sausage are highly processed meats that are high in saturated fat, calories and salt, making them nutritional problems. I don't recommend bacon or sausage with any breakfast—or at any other time.

Lunch and Supper Remarks

Lunch provides a nutritional boost in the middle of the day. It doesn't need to be a large meal, but this can vary. Some retired folks eat a good breakfast and have a large meal in early afternoon. They may have a small meal late in the day. If the meals are nutritionally sound, this pattern is fine.

We eat a light lunch at noon, followed by a hearty meal in the evening. Lunch usually consists of a large glass of blended vegetables or fruit, sometimes alone, or sometimes with soup or a sandwich. Fiber is preserved in blended veggie or fruit drinks, and they have great nutritional value. Juicers, unlike blenders, remove most of the fiber and roughage, producing a juice with less nutritional value.

Tastes are a factor in nutrition. Fruit juice, with its natural sweet taste, appeals to many people. The story is different with vegetable drinks, most of which are not naturally sweet. Getting used to their taste may take some adjustment. Yet, they have a vibrantly healthy kind of taste that is good when one's taste buds adjust to them. Blending various fruits and vegetables together often produces a tasty drink.

The mind is key in learning to enjoy new tastes. A genetic factor is involved in taste, but most food preferences are culturally determined. There is great variation in foods around the world. People like foods they are familiar with, but anyone can learn to appreciate new tastes if willing to make the effort. I've learned to enjoy a wide variety of foods from many areas of the world.

We have hearty suppers. Our meals are mainly plant-based, though we may eat fish once or twice a month. People sometimes think it's hard to plan meals without a meat entrée, but it's not. As with tastes, this is largely a matter of one's mindset. I became vegetarian in the early 1990s when accumulating evidence convinced me that avoiding meat was a healthier way to eat. We'd previously been trying vegetarian meals two or three days a week. This gradual approach toward healthier cuisine helped us succeed.

Our vegetarian diet was good, but I still recall my concern about how to plan meals without any meat. It turned out to be a non-issue. After we made the decision to stop eating meat, we learned to adapt to vegetarian meals and never looked back. We filled our dinner plates with a variety of colorful vegetables and greens, along with brown rice, potato, sweet potato, or some other vegetarian entrée, and we always left the dinner table satisfied and happy. Today, evidence supporting the plant-based way of eating is strong.[10]

The key to a healthy diet involves eating lots of vegetables, fruits and other wholesome foods. Meat doesn't have to be totally stopped for the sake

---

10. http://www.vegetarian-nutrition.info/updates/vegetarian_diets_health_benefits.php

of better health, but it's smart to limit red meat to less than three servings a week. One doesn't have to become a vegetarian to do this.

Inexpensive Costs of Eating Well

Many people think that a healthy diet is expensive when compared to the standard American diet. The answer is that it's not more expensive overall, but there are several aspects to this question worth examining.

When Marion Nestle did a cost analysis of fresh produce a few years ago, she found conventional fresh produce to be remarkably inexpensive per serving, costing "so little that even people on very low incomes could afford it." She concluded that cost is not really the barrier that keeps people from eating more vegetables and fruit.[11]

Organic fruits and vegetables are more expensive than their conventional counterparts, but this cost difference is coming down steadily, and is now small in many cases. As the organic produce sector keeps growing, its relative cost continues to drop.

Meat is a fairly expensive item in most grocery budgets. Reducing meat in the diet cuts this expense down, compensating for the cost of buying more organic produce. Solid research shows that billions of dollars can be saved nationally from lower health care costs connected with healthy diets.[12] Individuals can expect similar savings also.

On a global scale, traditional indigenous dietary patterns may be among the healthiest anyone can follow. Often consisting of local grains, beans, nuts and vegetables, with minimal amounts of meat, these are inexpensive. Healthy eating does not have to be costly. The simplest, least costly diets in

11. Marion Nestle. *What to Eat,* New York, NY: (North Point Press, 2006), p 63, 64.

12. Nicholson A Barnard ND, and JL Howard. "The Medical Costs Attributable to Meat Consumption." *Preventive Medicine* 1995; 24:646-55.

the world may also be the healthiest!

Healthy Zimbabwean Meals

The traditional Zimbabwean meal consisted of sadza, indigenous vegetables, greens and fruit, and a bit of meat on special occasions. Sadza is a thick cornmeal mash. Traditionally, it was made from roughly ground cornmeal, with all its fiber and micronutrients intact. Today most urban Zimbabweans buy refined cornmeal that has been stripped of fiber and many nutrients, just as with refined flour.

When I'm in Zimbabwe, I enjoy sadza with beans and veggies occasionally, but I prefer unrefined, or "rough" sadza, as it is made and served in rural areas. It's more nutritious than refined sadza, and I think it has more flavor. This traditional meal, combined with all the walking done by rural villagers, gives them a healthier lifestyle than is true for most modern urbanites.

During the months that I teach at Africa University, I cook most of my own meals in the Guest House where I stay. My breakfast usually consists of a fresh orange, hot oatmeal and raisin porridge topped with sliced banana, followed by a cup of African herbal tea (Rooibos), and a slice of whole wheat bread and jam on the side.

For lunch, I often have an avocado sandwich, consisting of half a ripe avocado spread between two slices of whole wheat bread. Alternatively, I have a peanut butter and banana sandwich that is easy to fix. I spread two tablespoons of locally-made peanut butter on a slice of whole wheat bread, add banana slices (sliced length-wise,) and top this with another slice of whole wheat bread. I usually eat a locally grown apple after my sandwich. This makes a delicious and nutritious lunch.

My supper is usually a big serving of brown rice mixed with baked beans and tomato sauce. I always have several cooked veggies on the side and a slice of plain whole wheat bread (no topping). Veggies vary, but usually consist of some combination of greens, butternut squash, fresh okra pods, broccoli, cauliflower, sweet potato, eggplant, carrots, beets, and/or cabbage. I may have a piece of fruit after this meal, but I'm often so full that I forego any dessert.

In summary, my diet in Zimbabwe is simple, but nutritious. I enjoy it very much. My goal is to have ten servings of veggies and fruit daily, and I usually make my goal. This diet is not expensive, contrary to the oft-expressed idea that a healthy diet is too expensive for most people. It's not!

What About Snacks, Desserts, and Eating Out?

Snacks, desserts, and eating out pose common nutritional pitfalls everywhere. Following are some ways they can be handled without falling into undesirable nutritional traps.

The best way to handle snacks is to substitute healthy snacks for unhealthy ones. There are a number of good options for this. A piece of fruit, such as an apple, an orange, or a plum makes a delicious snack that is nutritious and low in calories. Depending on the season, there are many other fruit choices that you can make, ranging from a piece of cantaloupe to a tangerine.

Another possibility is to have a fresh veggie snack such as carrot sticks, celery sticks, or a handful of grape tomatoes. These are also nutritious and low in calories. Other possibilities include a handful of nuts or a half-teaspoon of peanut butter on a multigrain saltine cracker. These are healthy choices but are higher in fat content and calories, so it's best not to overdo them.

Fruit-flavored yogurt snacks are sometimes suggested, but two drawbacks make them problematic. First, they are sweetened with sugar or a sugar substitute, which is not desirable. Second, yogurt is a dairy product that carries nutritional baggage. For these reasons, I do not suggest yogurt snacks as a rule.

A key point with regard to snacks is to avoid stocking up a lot of tempting but unhealthy snacks. If you have unhealthy snacks on hand, that is what you'll reach for. Keep a variety of healthy snacks available instead. Whatever is most convenient is what you're likely to indulge in.

A related point is to not stock any sodas or energy drinks at home. They are tempting to have for their claimed energy boost, but they have serious drawbacks. It's better to have a glass of water to quench your thirst. You can drink water alone or have it along with a healthy snack.

Desserts are a major pitfall for many people. The problem with most conventional desserts is that they are loaded with sugar and fat. This combination is deadly in the long term, but cake, cookies, pie, ice cream, and a host of other desserts are too tempting for many to resist. What is the best way of getting around this pitfall in a healthy way?

One of the best ways is to enjoy fruit for dessert. Fruit is delicious and nutritious, and it satisfies the sweet tooth that often needs soothing. When we have dessert at home, we usually have fruit. We often share an apple after lunch, and we may have cantaloupe, honeydew, oranges, organic grapes, watermelon, tangerines, or some other fruit for dessert after supper. Fresh fruit is always good, and it never leaves us feeling bloated.

If you're a guest where a rich, sugar-laden dessert has been prepared for festive occasions such as Christmas or to celebrate a special occasion, one option is to ask for a small serving or to split it with your partner. A small overdose of sugar won't destroy your health, but be careful not to let it slip into ever more frequent exceptions.

After a filling meal, there may be no need for dessert. We often skip dessert after supper to simply enjoy a cup of hot herbal tea. Skipping an unhealthy dessert is always a smart option.

Eating out is perhaps the most dangerous pitfall of all, because hidden traps are found everywhere in most restaurant meals. Excessive salt, sugar, and hidden fat are the rule in most fast food meals, and they're prevalent even in prestigious restaurants. Yet, eating out has become common. Almost 50 percent of meals served in America are now restaurant or take-out meals. What are healthy options?

The first and perhaps smartest option is to skip going out, and eat more home-cooked meals. Statistics show that people eat more healthfully when they prepare their food at home. Still, eating out on occasion is enjoyable, so what are the best options then? The answer is to avoid most fast food outlets and make choices as healthfully as possible wherever you eat.

To summarize the difficult issue of eating out, the best solution is to eat home-cooked meals most of the time. When you do eat out, avoid most fast food places, and make your food orders as wisely as possible wherever you choose to eat.

Vitamins

Do vitamins and other supplements contribute to good health? This issue deserves a chapter or book of its own, but I will summarize it as briefly and accurately as possible.

After vitamins were first discovered and isolated, they seemed like miraculous healing agents, and indeed they were. When a specific vitamin matched a specific deficiency, the cure was dramatic. As a result, vitamins gained a reputation of being miracle health factors, and many people began pushing vitamins as cure-alls for everything.

Today we know that vitamins are only a tiny fraction of the healing spectrum provided by whole foods. Most plants have thousands of anti-oxidants and phytochemicals, as well as fiber and minerals. All of these micronutrients are valuable for good health.

Multivitamin capsules have a few dozen vitamins and minerals at most. They cannot include the thousands of valuable nutrients carried in whole foods. This means that anyone who rarely eats veggies and fruit is missing many vital nutrients. It is impossible to make up for their loss, even by taking a handful of vitamins every day.

We also know that vitamin megadoses can be unhealthy. Scientists once thought large doses of certain vitamins might help prevent some kinds of disease. When this was tested in large-scale studies involving thousands of people, many vitamins were linked to an increased risk of disease rather than providing any protection.

What all this means is that vitamins are valuable nutrients within the whole foods where they are naturally found. They are less valuable when extracted as isolated factors from those foods. With overuse as isolated extracts, they may even cause harm.

Are vitamins ever a good idea to prevent disease? Yes! It's a good idea for pregnant women to take multivitamins to prevent certain birth defects in their babies. We know that folic acid deficiency during pregnancy is associated with a risk of serious neural tube defects in newborns. Folic acid is especially abundant in green leafy vegetables, but young women who don't eat many vegetables need folic acid supplementation.

Vitamins are also a good idea for babies and small children until they are old enough to eat a well-rounded, wholesome diet. However, if parents are good models for eating a wholesome diet, children can learn to do this at a young age.

Vitamin B-12 is the only vitamin that is found almost exclusively in meat or animal products like eggs and milk. Because of this, strict vegans should take a B-12 pill daily.

Vitamin D, the "sunshine vitamin," is deficient in many people who do not get adequate exposure to sunlight. There is increasing evidence that vitamin D has greater value for a variety of conditions than we knew in the past. People in northern climates and shut-ins should take it daily. A dose of 1000 units daily is safe for most adults.

Some health experts suggest taking a daily multivitamin as a kind of health insurance for all adults. Is there any benefit in doing this? When this question was tested in large-scale studies carried out for years, no significant difference was found between those who took multivitamins and those who took none.[13] Another recent study suggested that daily multivitamins may carry some benefit, so the jury is still out on this.

In summary, people who take multivitamins must not fool themselves into thinking it will make up for poor eating habits. Evidence to support taking multivitamins to insure good health is lacking. Eating an abundance of wholesome food with well-balanced meals is more valuable than any vitamin pill can possibly be. I don't take multivitamins, much preferring the option of eating lots of good food.

Nutritional Fitness Summary

Consuming enough calories to meet one's energy needs is not the same as achieving good nutritional fitness. It's important to eat enough food to avoid malnutrition, but overeating is also a cause of serious health problems. Taking vitamins does not correct for poor nutrition, as I've noted above. So how does one become nutritionally fit?

---

13. "NIH State-of-the-Science Conference Statement on Multivitamin/Mineral Supplements and Chronic Disease Prevention". NIH Consens State Sci Statements 23 (2) 2006, 1–30.

Optimal nutritional health comes from maintaining a good balance of macronutrients (carbohydrate, fats, and proteins) and micronutrients (antioxidants, minerals, and vitamins.) This helps maintain one's body in good nutritional shape, free of too much fat, sugar, cholesterol, or other elements where they're not needed. Unfortunately, this kind of fitness is not common in America today.

Even if people look like the picture of health, they can have atherosclerosis of the arteries, a very unhealthy condition. We know this arterial disease is widespread in America by the teenage years, often becoming life-threatening by mid-life.[14] Too much body fat is not good for health either. Unfortunately, obesity and atherosclerosis are both epidemic in the West today.

One becomes nutritionally fit by eating wholesome foods in abundance while avoiding foods that undermine health. Healthy meals should include six to ten servings of fruits and vegetables daily. Nine or ten servings a day provide optimal benefit. Yet, the average American eats less than three servings a day, showing how far short of the mark we fall when it comes to nutritional fitness.

It's not difficult to get in at least six servings of fruits and veggies a day. We did that even before we became vegetarian. Two servings for breakfast (orange juice and a banana), two for lunch (salad and a fruit), and two or three for supper (salad and two or three veggies), add up to six or seven for the day. That is easy to achieve if one makes a point of doing so. Making this a consistent habit is not hard.

Leafy greens are one of nature's most nutritious treasures. The book, *Leafy Greens*, is a great source of recipes for over 30 kinds of greens.[15] We enjoy raw greens (like Romaine lettuce, spinach greens, or baby spring

14. http://jama.ama-assn.org/content/281/8/727.full

15. Mark Bittman. *Leafy Greens*, (New York, NY: Macmillan, 1995).

greens) in our salads most days, and we have a serving of steamed or lightly cooked greens of one type or another with our supper most evenings. They are wonderful.

Nutritional fitness is not the only pillar needed to support good health, but it is one in need of serious attention, as shown by the epidemic of nutritionally-related diseases sweeping around the world. Lack of sound nutrition is a major factor in obesity, type 2 diabetes, coronary artery disease, hypertension, stroke, and others. The commitment to create and eat healthy meals is a major key to healthy living.

Recipes for Healthy Living is a good resource that can be found on my website. These simple nutritious recipes come from my wife Carol and me, as well as from Rand and Colleen Dodge. Well-tested by the authors, these recipes promote healthy living.

In the paragraphs below, Randall offers good practical tips for creating healthy meals.

Practical Tips (by Rand)

Simplicity in eating has been a key part of my health journey. I try to eat two-thirds of my total calories in fresh vegetables, whole grains, and fruits. That means I start each day with whole-grain cereal loaded with fresh fruit.

For breakfast I typically have oatmeal or shredded wheat with at least three servings of fresh seasonal fruit. Blueberries, blackberries, raspberries, strawberries, bananas, peaches, cooked apples, and more can be combined to deliver a delicious and healthy jump-start to each new day. In my attempt to cut back on dairy products, I have experimented with several alternatives to skim milk. Soy milk and rice milk are options I tried but I have settled on unsweetened almond milk. To me, it is the most satisfying and offers some nutritional benefits as well.

Then I usually have two cups of vegetable soup for lunch, along with a dozen baby carrots that I sometimes dip in a little hummus. We (my wife and I) make a big pot of fresh soup on the weekend and then store it in the refrigerator in two-cup sealable containers. It is then easy to grab a container of soup and snack bag of carrots to take to work with me. Each week the soup is a little different but all of our soups have lots of fresh onions, leeks, kale, spinach, carrots, peas, corn, and peppers. Some weeks we add dried lentils or beans. Then we flavor it with fresh herbs or ground spices. It is a wonderful way to refuel during the middle of the day.

Dinner is almost always a huge salad! And every salad is unique! We start with fresh romaine or spinach, adding beet greens or Swiss chard or field greens to the mixing bowl. Then we start adding chopped onions, celery, grated carrots or beets, chopped sweet peppers, sliced tomatoes, homemade black bean and corn salsa, couscous, sliced raw almonds, and a little ground flax seed. We also love to add some fruit to our salad. Berries add a nice sweet flavor and mix well with the other ingredients. Finally, we make our own salad dressings. One of our favorites is balsamic vinegar mixed with lemon or lime juice along with a little olive oil and honey and seasoned with just a touch of soy sauce or hot sauce. Sometimes we will also mix some dry herbs or Mrs. Dash in the dressing.

To supplement the large salad, we usually have one or two cooked vegetables on the side or even added to the salad. Oven roasted Brussels sprouts with chopped onions and mushrooms make great salad toppings! Fresh corn-on-the-cob or grilled squash make great side dishes. Most days we don't eat any meat but once or twice each week we will have a small quantity of fish with dinner. Grilled salmon goes well with salad or we sometimes open a small can of tuna packed in water. Whether we add protein or not, we never leave the dinner table hungry!

As for snacks, I typically have a piece of fruit mid-morning and mid-afternoon. Occasionally I'll make a fruit smoothie on the weekend or air pop some popcorn if we are playing games in the evening.

Preparing food like this takes a little more time than just popping something in the microwave. But we find the rewards worth it. My wife and I enjoy making soups and salads together. We also enjoy gardening together and relishing the fresh produce from our garden. All the organic waste from our food preparation goes into a compost tumbler and then back to our garden. And we've cut back significantly on watching television which was a far less valuable use of our time than gardening and exercising. Although we are still busy, our lives are simpler than they used to be. The bottom line is that we feel better and are less stressed.

CHAPTER EIGHT

The Dreadful "Sitting Disease"

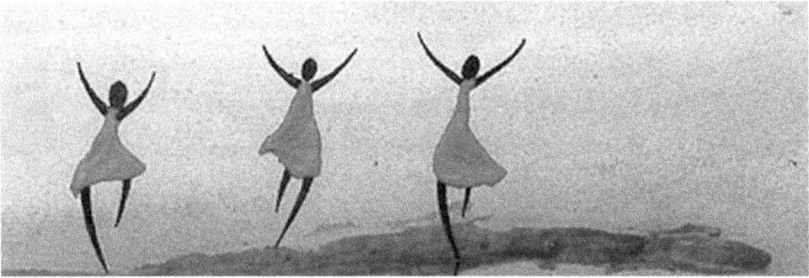

Adam, like many people, has a desk job that involves sitting most of the workday. The combination of TV and a laptop computer at home means that Adam sits most of the time at home also. Of course, going anywhere is almost always by car. Adam's sedentary lifestyle provides little allowance for any physical activity. In this chapter we'll take a look at the health hazards connected with lack of adequate physical activity. We'll find out why it's important to avoid the "Sitting Disease."

Sedentary Living Common Today

Being inactive is harmful for the body's normal functions. Our bodies were designed for vigorous activity. Most people realize that exercise is important, but many fail to get the exercise their bodies need. Computers and television are so common now that many people are sedentary both at work and play. Instead of being physically active during their free time, millions of people sit at home or at sports bars to watch highly paid athletes, entertainers, and media personalities perform for them. Since sedentary living is so common, let's look at its risks.

Problems of Sedentary Living

Beyond losing the benefits that come from exercise, sedentary life imposes its own costs on health. Sedentary people pay a high price in terms of the gradual deterioration of health triggered by inactivity. Eventually, this also leads to high medical costs. The link between inactivity and poor health is often overlooked because it develops so slowly, but with long-term statistical analysis, an increased risk of serious health problems like heart disease, type 2 diabetes, obesity, and certain kinds of cancer is clearly related to length of daily sitting time.

Two terms are worth defining before going into the problems of sedentary living. Anabolism is the process of building up or renewing body tissues. Catabolism is the process of tearing down and removing damaged cells from the body. Both processes are vitally important because we are continuously building up and tearing down tissues in our bodies.

When you burn your tongue by drinking anything that's too hot, the injured cells are torn down and removed by means of catabolism. New cells and taste buds are quickly rebuilt, and within a day or two, your burned tongue is healed. Both the catabolic and anabolic processes are essential to accomplish this task. These same processes work continuously to keep every body part in good shape. This enables us to function at optimum efficiency—as long as both processes are working effectively.

When we exercise regularly, we help both processes work well. When we don't exercise, we lose much of the stimulus needed to renew tissues. The muscles are the main sites where rejuvenating proteins called cytokines are made. The best stimulus to making them is exercise. Exercise is a key to boosting the rebuilding cytokines and get them circulating to every part of the body.[15]

When we fail to exercise, we don't get this strong boost. Worse yet, inactivity fosters indolent catabolic processes. The paradoxical result is that our bodies "wear out" more quickly from sedentary living than from energetic lifestyles. After riding in a car for several hours, I feel stiff when I first get out. This clears up only after I stir around enough to get my muscles and joints loosened up. Yet I can walk miles without feeling stiff. In a real sense, movement "lubricates"our bodies. Our cardiovascular, nervous, and musculoskeletal systems are all energized by movement. Without movement, the tissues in our bodies tend to gel and eventually lead to premature aging.

It's been well established for years that regular exercise helps prevent complications of a sedentary lifestyle. More recent research from Australia and the USA suggests that sitting more than four to six hours a day poses increased health risks, even when subjects are getting some exercise. One or more enzymes activated by physical activity seem to shut down after four hours of sitting, leading to greater risk of developing higher blood sugar, blood pressure, abdominal fat, and abnormal cholesterol.

The Sitting Disease

The evidence for the constellation of health problems connected with prolonged sitting is so strong that it is now being called the Sitting Disease. Although this is not an official diagnosis, the term is being used by many physicians, including those in medical institutions such as the Mayo Clinic. There is even concern that some complications of the *Sitting Disease* may develop in people who exercise daily if they sit for too many hours without

---

15. Chris Crowley and Henry S. Lodge, MD. *Younger Next Year*, (New York, NY: Workman Publishing, 2004).

activity during the rest of the day.[16]

I sit at my computer for six to eight hours several days a week as I write this book, meaning that I'm vulnerable to the *Sitting Disease* even though I also exercise faithfully for 30 to 60 minutes a day. This exercise is valuable, but it's important to break up long hours of sitting by taking brief exercise breaks every hour or so. Physical activity reduces risks and makes life healthier. We'll discuss this in more detail in Chapters Nine and Ten.

Sedentary Living and Obesity

Unfortunately, sedentary living is also linked to obesity in a catch-22 kind of situation. Sedentary people may eat as many calories as more active people, but burn up less of them. The end result is a tendency to gain excess weight. The more weight they gain, the less they exercise, and the heavier they become. The heavier they get, the less they want to exercise. Eventually, this vicious cycle throws them into the obesity crunch that characterizes so much of the Western world today.

For someone trapped in obesity, escaping is like trying to climb out of quicksand. It's as if fat calories won't let go. Escaping obesity is a challenge, but it's possible. Still, it's better to avoid the obesity quagmire in the first place. Adopting a healthy lifestyle at an early age is a good strategy. Parents who help their children do this give them a great start in life. The most effective way of teaching children a healthy lifestyle is to model it. Parents need to be as dedicated to physical activity as they want their children to be.

This is not a minor issue (even though it involves minors!) According to the CDC, childhood obesity has more than doubled in the past 30 years, going from seven percent in 1980 to nearly 18 percent in 2010, while adolescent obesity (ages 12-19) has tripled from five percent to 18 percent in

---

16. http://www.mayoclinic.com/health/sitting-disease/MY02177; http://www.cdc.gov/healthyyouth/obesity/facts.htm

that same time. In 2010, more than one third of all children and adolescents were overweight or obese.

The health implications of these statistics are disturbing, both for the children at risk and for our national health. Obese youth are much more likely to be at risk of heart disease as adults, with 70 percent of them having at least one risk factor for heart disease. They are also more likely to have prediabetes, and are at greater risk of type 2 diabetes, heart disease, stroke, osteoarthritis and several types of cancer as adults. Physical inactivity is a big factor in setting the stage for these problems to develop.

In conclusion, the *Sitting Disease* is a serious problem. The long-term health outlook for those with this disease is dreadful. In Chapters Nine and Ten, we'll look at the lifelong benefits of physical activity. If it's not a regular part of your life, it needs to be. We'll discuss how to bring it into your life as a continuing source of joy.

CHAPTER NINE

The Awesome Benefits of Physical Activity

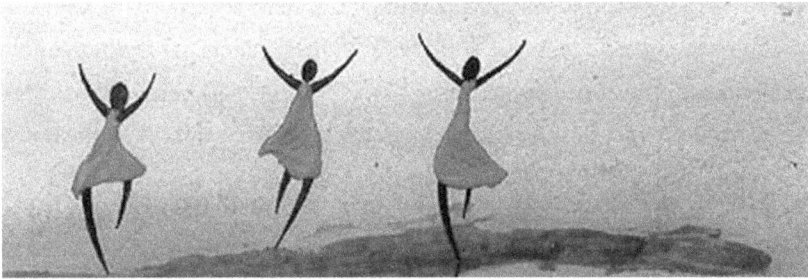

Adam, like most people, realizes that exercise is good for health. Yet, even after learning about the hazards of the sedentary life, Adam finds it hard to maintain an exercise program. In this chapter, we look at some of the pros and cons about physical activity. There are a few cons, mainly due to poor judgment, but they are outweighed by its awesome benefits. Adam learns why these benefits are so impressive as we explore this subject.

The Power of Exercise

Physical activity is essential for healthy living. Our bodies were designed for vigorous activity. Most people realize that exercise is important, but many fail to get the exercise their bodies need. How does exercise enhance health? Muscles need exercise to maintain strength, but exercising does much more than tone up your muscles. A good level of exercise helps every cell in your body from your brain cells to your tiptoes, and everything in between. It's also good for mental health. Many studies show that regular exercise is good for patients with depression and other mental disorders.

Regular exercise promotes good health, but beyond that, it helps keep our bodies functionally younger than they would be otherwise. We know this from much careful research on the physiology of exercise. The book, *Younger Next Year*, by Chris Crowley and Henry Lodge, MD, summarizes a few of these research findings in a way that's easy to understand.[17]

The muscles are the main sites where rejuvenating proteins called cytokines are made. The best stimulus to making them is exercise. In addition to promoting these cytokines, exercise substantially increases the blood flow through your muscles. This increased blood flow picks up rejuvenating cytokines from the muscles and carries them to every tissue and cell in the body.

The result is that every cell in the body gets a renewal stimulus every time you exercise. If you do this regularly, your body becomes functionally younger than it was before you started exercising regularly. The key requirement is to exercise 30 minutes or more a day, six days a week.

Types of Exercise

There are many kinds of exercise that can be done, and all of them have some benefit. For most people, the easiest kind of exercise to do is walking. When done regularly, simple walking is an excellent form of exercise. Although its value is often underestimated, walking is the most time-proven physical activity known to man. It has been the main way people have moved throughout history. Today, we know that it is also one of the most effective forms of exercise we can perform.

One of the advantages of walking is that it requires no special equipment beyond a good pair of walking shoes. Other advantages are that you can find good places to walk almost anywhere, and it is something you can do alone or with friends.

---

17. Chris Crowley and Henry S. Lodge, MD. *Younger Next Year*, (New York, NY: Workman Publishing, 2004).

In *Younger Next Year*, John is a man who retired at age 65 with serious health problems. He was one hundred pounds overweight, had high cholesterol and high blood pressure, and was in generally poor shape.

Although he didn't like exercise in any form, he reluctantly agreed to walk on the beach once a day, six days a week. (The home he retired to in Florida was only one block from the beach.) At first he could barely walk one hundred yards, and that exhausted him, but within a few months he was walking one mile a day and feeling much better.

By the end of a year, he was walking five miles a day. He had lost 60 pounds. His cholesterol and blood pressure were normal, and he felt great. According to Crowley, John looked ten years younger. It was not easy for John to begin his walking program, but he did it, and because he stayed with it, he reaped its benefits.

There are other benefits to walking besides burning calories and helping with weight control. Because it is a weight-bearing exercise, it helps keep bones strong and healthy. Osteoporosis and bone fractures are much less common among people who walk regularly than among sedentary Americans.

Walking is more universal than any other kind of exercise, but there are many other helpful kinds of physical activity. Jogging, bicycling, swimming, dancing, clogging, running, tennis, jump-roping, rowing, kayaking, canoeing, cross-country skiing, and stair-stepping are a few popular kinds of aerobic exercise that can be done.

Jane is a 78-year old woman who combines walking and bicycling. She walks two miles a day at least three days a week. She and her 80-year old husband also bicycle 20 to 50 miles several days a week. Once a year they do a "Century Ride," consisting of riding one hundred miles in a single day. Needless to say, they are remarkably fit!

Beyond its musculoskeletal benefits, aerobic exercise is good for the lungs and the cardiovascular system. It is good for the digestive system, the brain and the nervous system, and for mental, emotional, and physical health. It boosts the immune system and the health of every part of the body. It is a miraculous health tonic, and it is free!

In addition to aerobic exercise, there are two other basic types of exercise that are beneficial. Resistance exercise is commonly done in gyms with weight-lifting or resistance kinds of equipment. Body-building enthusiasts are noted for engaging in this type of exercise. In moderation, it's helpful for nearly everyone.

Flexibility exercises such as yoga, pilates [pill-ah'-tease] or tai-chi have also proven helpful for many people. They are worthwhile for people of all ages, and their popularity continues to grow steadily. Pilates combines some of the values and benefits of both flexibility and resistance training.

Problems Connected with Exercise

There are a few potential downsides to regular exercise. The first is trying to do too much too soon, leading to problems ranging from blisters and strained muscles to more serious injuries. "Weekend warriors" are vulnerable to this kind of injury. The key to preventing such injuries is to start any exercise program at a fairly low level of intensity, and then build it up gradually, but steadily.

It's important to start slowly in many kinds of exercise. It may be wise to see your doctor to get medical clearance for some of these exercises. A trainer to guide your pace and level of exercise can be a big help. Once you achieve a moderate level of exercise, you can often proceed at your own pace, always remembering not to step it up too rapidly.

A second potential downside is straining to reach lofty goals for which you are not ready. Paradoxically, this is a risk for seasoned exercisers who may over-strain in trying to reach high goals. This is a variant of trying to do too much too soon. The key to prevention is a careful training program and patience in pacing oneself.

A third pitfall is viewing exercise as a total health panacea. Some exercise enthusiasts believe in it so strongly that they neglect other crucial aspects of healthy living. An example is the exercise devotee who fails to follow a healthy diet, believing that exercise will protect him from any dietary excesses. The reality is that exercise and healthy eating are both important. Neglect of either one is foolish at best, and life-threatening at worst.

Jim Fixx was seriously overweight and a heavy smoker at age 35 when he began jogging in 1967. When he took up running, he quit smoking, and he went on to become a marathon runner. In 1977 he wrote *The Complete Book of Running*. It became an international best-seller that was known as the running "bible" for serious runners. The book made him famous, and he was widely viewed as being someone who had reached the epitome of fitness.

However, Fixx had other risk factors that he reportedly neglected, evidently thinking that exercise was his guarantee of good health. It wasn't. Even though he was as physically fit as anyone could be, he dropped dead during a training run in 1984. He had suffered a massive heart attack. An autopsy showed that all his coronary arteries were severely diseased, apparently related to unhealthy eating choices. Exercise alone does not guarantee optimal health!

His story emphasizes the lesson that nutritional fitness goes hand-in-hand with physical fitness. Neither of these pillars of health stands alone. Together, they provide stronger support for good health than either one does by itself. This kind of reinforcement is true for all the principles of good health. Because of such mutually reinforcing effects, an overall healthy lifestyle is more beneficial than any single kind of fitness by itself.

A quick review of cardiovascular function helps makes it clear why nutrition and exercise are both crucial for optimal health. At rest, the heart beats about 100,000 times each day, pumping five liters of blood per minute (2,000 gallons a day) through 60,000 miles of blood vessels in the adult human body. With moderately intense exercise, the amount of blood being pumped around the circulatory system goes up to about 20 liters per minute. Seventy percent of this blood flow goes to exercising muscles that need much more oxygen during exercise.[18]

Obviously, the heart is a very hard-working organ. When one considers that it works for up to a hundred years or more without a break, one's respect for this awesome organ has to be great. The value of regular exercise is two-fold for the heart. Research studies show that regular exercise strengthens the heart beat, making it more efficient, and allowing it to slow down at rest. In regular exercisers, the resting heart rate often drops to less than 60 beats a minute, saving the heart nearly 20,000 heart beats over a 24-hour period. This adds years of potential good heart function.

A second way in which exercise helps the heart is that other working muscles literally assist blood and lymphatic flow back to the heart. This booster effect by exercising muscles eases the heart's workload, giving it the potential of longer life expectancy.

Wholesome nutrition also has a favorable impact on the heart and circulatory system. As mentioned in chapter five, highly refined or processed foods and those high in saturated fat are damaging in their effect on the heart and circulatory system. These foods are the main contributing causes to serious atherosclerosis of arteries, the "pipelines" that deliver fuel and oxygen to every vital organ, and ultimately to every tissue and cell in the body.

Severe atherosclerotic plaques throughout the arterial tree damage the elasticity and strength of arterial walls, while also causing obstructions to

---

18. Dean Hodgkin. *Physiology and Fitness*, (Chantilly, Virginia: *The Great Courses*, Number 1960) DVD.

blood flow through these vital "pipelines." Such obstructions can block up to 95 percent of the free flow of blood. The extra work required of the heart to pump blood against high pressure through miles of obstructing pipelines makes one realize the key value of keeping these blood vessels clean.

This helps clarify why wholesome nutrition and healthy exercise are both important to good health. Both are essential for the health and performance of the heart and entire circulatory system that is so vital to the health of all other organs, tissues and cells in the body. When they realize this, most people want to have a healthy heart pumping blood throughout a healthy arterial system to maintain the health of their entire body. Wholesome nutrition and healthy exercise are both crucial to achieving this goal.

A final potential downside to exercise is the risk of becoming an exercise addict. Someone who puts exercise ahead of all else in life may be an addict. While this isn't a danger for most of us, a few people go overboard with their commitment to exercise, sacrificing quality family time and much else to their exercise compulsion. For most people, the risk of exercising too much pales in comparison to the risks of sedentary living.

What About People Who Can't Exercise?

A final question concerns people who are unable to exercise because of serious illness or severe disability. What can they do? This is a significant issue, but in most cases it's not insurmountable. People with disability can exercise.

The International Paralympic Committee plans the Paralympics that follow the Olympic games every four years. They have grown steadily in importance and recognition over the years, with over 3,900 athletes participating in the 2008 Summer Paralympic Games in Beijing. Athletes with amputations, blindness, cerebral palsy, and other disabilities are now involved in a wide variety of sporting events, including wheelchair events for paraplegics.

The Special Olympics are athletic events for intellectually impaired people, such as those with Down Syndrome. Like the Paralympics, they have grown in recognition over the years since being founded in 1968. Both have inspired many disabled people to get involved in physical activities. The main point here is that disability does not disqualify people from healthy exercise.

What about the very elderly? They can exercise if encouraged to do so. Adult Living Facilities usually schedule an hour every weekday for chair exercises. Even patients in wheelchairs can participate in them. Mild flexibility and strength exercises are included, and they have proven to be very beneficial for the elderly. Even at one-hundred years of age, my father looked forward to this daily activity every day when he was in an ALF.

People who are hospitalized with severe injuries or illnesses may be unable to exercise, but even in these situations, physical therapy usually proves to be helpful. Patients who have major surgery, including cardiac surgery, are often started on physical therapy the very next day. The first day may simply involve being helped out of bed or with taking a few steps away from the bed, but it's a start. Each day, the therapist guides the patient in ever-longer walks.

This quick survey of the impact of exercise on health should convince even the most skeptical readers that exercise is an important part of healthy living. The big question is what you can do to actively integrate exercise into your daily life. The next chapter is dedicated to helping you do this.

CHAPTER TEN

A Simple Plan to Be Physically Active

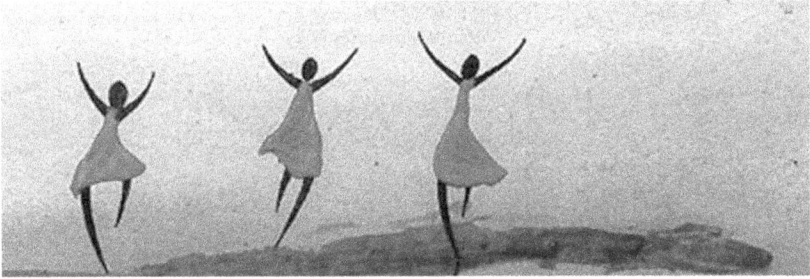

After learning about the awesome benefits of exercise, Adam decides it's too valuable to keep neglecting. Still, when it's not a basic necessity, it's tough to make exercise a regular part of one's life. How does one do this? A simple plan to get started helps. When regular exercise begins to kick in as a valued experience, commitment becomes easier. That's when Adam becomes an exercise cheerleader!

The Value of a Pedometer

I have carried a pedometer in my pocket for the last ten years. This simple but valuable tool for walkers and runners tells me how many steps I have taken at the end of each day. It does other things also, but keeping track of my steps is what I value most.

The reason it helps is two-fold. First, knowing the number of steps I take each day is the best way to know how well I'm doing with my exercise goal. My daily step count gives me my score for the day. The key to keeping score is my pedometer. Following is my step-scoring system.

Grade for Number of Steps per Day

1000 - 1999 steps = F

2000 - 3999 steps = D

4000 - 5999 steps = C

6000 - 7999 steps = B

8000 - 9999 steps = A

10,000 or more steps is Superlative

My goal is to take at least 6,000 steps a day, which is equivalent to a "B" in this grading system. If I get 8,000 or more steps (an "A"), I'm happy with my day. If I get between 4,000 to 6,000 steps, it is a mediocre day. If I get less than 4,000 steps, I'm doing very poorly and know that I must do better the next day.

I'm not obsessive-compulsive about this grading system. I devised it to help anyone understand what the step-count means, but I don't ever write it down. I simply glance at the pedometer before going to bed to get a quick idea of how I did that day, and this helps me set my goal for the next day. Simple though this system is, it's powerfully motivating, and that is the second value of my pedometer.

A quick comment about the 10,000 step level: Many exercise enthusiasts recommend setting a daily goal of at least 10,000 steps a day. While that's ideal if you can do it, in my view it's not a realistic goal for many people. To take 10,000 steps is equal to about five miles for the average walker (2,000 steps is about one mile.)

There have been weeks when I averaged over 10,000 steps a day, but that's usually on vacations when I can hike to my heart's content. It's great when I can do this, and I thoroughly enjoy those long hikes, but they are not my typical weeks. Most weeks I average between six to nine thousand steps a day, hitting ten thousand steps only once a week or so, and that's OK.

Many people don't have the luxury of devoting 90 minutes or more to exercise daily. From a health standpoint, it's not necessary to do so. Good research studies show that people get good benefits from exercising 30 to 60 minutes a day. Even 15 minutes a day provides some benefit, but about 45 minutes of exercise daily seems to provide optimal health benefits. If you time your exercise, 45 minutes daily is a good goal.

A Simple Exercise Plan for Good Health

Most people can find 30 minutes a day to devote to exercise if they truly believe it's important. Often, this is simply a matter of giving exercise the high priority that it deserves in their lives. Spending 30 minutes doing healthy exercise provides much more value than 30 minutes spent watching most TV programs.

Following is a simple plan for anyone who wishes to begin a regular exercise program. This is a two-tiered plan. The first tier is very simple, designed for anyone who has zero fitness, but wants to start an exercise program. It's appropriate for almost anyone, but if you have any medical problem requiring medical supervision, please get clearance from your doctor before starting the plan. If you feel reasonably fit, you can start off with Tier Two, but if any doubt exists about your level of fitness, it's best to begin with Tier One.

Walking plan pre-requisites:

1. A good pair of walking shoes. You can buy specific walking shoes, or you can use a pair you already own if they fit well and are comfortable to walk in. A good comfortable fit is very important!

2. Comfortable clothes suitable for the prevailing weather.

3. A good walking surface and environment. If you have good sidewalks or paths in your neighborhood, that is often the best place to walk. If you don't have a good place to walk at home, a nearby park may be a good choice. Many malls allow walkers in their corridors before stores open. A final option is to use a treadmill at home or at a nearby gym. Wherever you choose to walk, it's important that it be safe, convenient, and easy to use.

4. A calendar. Plan your month in advance and write down your starting walk-time on your calendar every day. This is more important than you realize. You are making an exercise appointment, and writing it down firms it up in your mind as well as on your calendar.

Walking Schedule

Week One: Walk **five minutes** daily for five or six days. You decide on the time of day best for you.

Week Two: Walk **ten minutes** daily for five or six days. Walk at a modest pace. Don't worry about distance.

Week Three: Walk **15 minutes** daily for five or six days. You are making good progress.

Week Four: Walk **20 minutes** daily for five or six days.

Week Five: Walk **25 minutes** daily for five or six days. You are doing well. Keep up the good work!

Week Six: Walk **30 minutes** daily for five or six days. Congratulations!

You have completed Tier One of the basic exercise plan! Tier Two adds more distance and a bit of variety into the plan, but walking remains the mainstay of the program.

Tier Two continues a walking schedule, but adds optional resistance exercises twice a week. These exercises involve moving weights in a variety of ways. Complete discussion of resistance training is beyond the scope of this book, but it's worth noting that resistance exercise, done in combination with endurance exercise, is valuable for health.

Resistance exercises are done in repetitive sets, with rest periods between the sets. The amount of resistance, or weight, is gradually increased over time. This kind of training can be done at home with simple weights, but for many people, gyms are the best place to do this kind of work. Beginners should have an experienced person or a trainer guide them in these exercises at first. Resistance training is often done two or three times a week, with off-days in between to allow stressed muscles to recuperate.

In the Tier Two schedule shown below, the resistance exercises are suggested twice a week. Please note that these resistance exercises are optional. If it's not possible for you to do them, simply continue the walking schedule. Walking a mile at a slow pace takes about 30 minutes; a moderate pace about 20 minutes; and a rapid pace about 15 minutes. If you can walk with a friend, that always seems to make the time fly by faster.

Week One: The walking schedule is increased a bit, and optional resistance exercises are added twice a week.

Monday—Walk **40 minutes** at a moderate pace, equivalent to walking two miles.

Tuesday—Walk **30 minutes** and do optional resistance exercises for 15 minutes with a trainer.

Wednesday—Walk **40 minutes** at a moderate pace.

Thursday—Walk **40 minutes** at a moderate pace.

Friday—Walk **40 minutes** at a moderate pace.

Saturday—Walk **30 minutes** at a moderate pace and do optional resistance exercises for **15 minutes**.

Sunday—Rest day. (A leisurely walk is always okay if you wish.)

Week Two: The resistance workout is optional. If you skip this, increase your walking to 45 minutes every day.

Monday—Walk **45 minutes** at a moderately fast pace.

Tuesday—Walk **20 minutes** and work out at the gym for **25 minutes**.

Wednesday—Walk **45 minutes** at a moderately fast pace.

Thursday—Walk **45 minutes** at a moderately fast pace.

Friday—Walk **45 minutes** at a moderately fast pace.

Saturday—Walk **20 minute**s and work out at the gym for **30 minutes**.

Sunday—Rest day. (A leisurely walk is OK if you wish.)

Weeks Three and Four—Same schedule as Week Two, except increase your gym workout time to 40 minutes, twice a week. If you skip the resistance exercises at the gym, increase your walking time to 45 minutes every day.

When you finish Tier Two, you will have completed ten weeks of exercises that contribute greatly to your health and your sense of well-being. Daily exercise of 45 minutes is the level that provides optimal benefit. At this point, you can branch into other kinds of exercise (we'll discuss the benefits of variety in exercise below.) Alternatively, you may simply continue your walking program at this level. Done consistently, it will enhance your health more than you may believe possible.

ABE for Fitness

A fairly new exercise program has been devised for people who have such busy schedules that they can't free up even 30 minutes a day for exercise. It's also a helpful way to add brief exercise breaks to anyone's day. As we noted in chapter eight, prolonged sitting is a hazard even for people who get some regular exercise. This program takes brief intervals of time as short as three or four minutes, and turns them into exercise opportunities throughout the day.

The ABE for Fitness program was created by Stephan Esser, MD, David Katz, MD, and members of the Harvard Institute of Lifestyle Medicine. ABE stands for Activity Bursts Everywhere. These consist of three to eight minute bursts of activity that anyone can take time to do at home, at work, or in any waiting kind of situation. Doing several of the quick ABE exercises daily will contribute to a good level of fitness.

An ABE website is available as a resource. It has a library of three to eight minute videos that demonstrate various kinds of activity bursts that can be done in various settings. I'm providing the link to this website with the consent of Dr. Esser.[19] If you're not able to devote a 30 to 60 minute block of time to exercise daily, I encourage you to take advantage of the ABE concept to build a good level of exercise into your life.

Additional Exercise Tips

Make your exercise time a fun part of your life. This is one of the most useful tips I have for you. If you can apply this single suggestion, it will greatly improve your chances of succeeding with your exercise program. Making exercise an integral part of your life depends on this more than anything else. If you don't enjoy what you do, you're not likely to keep it up.

But, someone will object: "How can you turn a boring exercise experience into a fun time?" There are many ways of doing this. I'll draw on my own experiences to illustrate some ways of making exercise fun, and I'll

---

19. http://www.abeforfitness.com/

start with basic walking.

I'm a morning person, and I usually take a two or three-mile walk at dawn. We live in a neighborhood on the north side of San Antonio, just where the hill country begins. I have several routes through our neighborhood, and I choose a different one each morning. In addition to observing a variety of things along the way, it's always interesting to see what has changed since I walked that way a week or so before. This morning I saw a deer with her two fawns just two blocks from our home. They looked at me as I approached, and then one of the fawns bolted across the street just ahead of me. The doe and the other fawn simply waited until I passed, and then they slowly sauntered across the street also.

A few blocks further on, I noticed a buzzard sitting on a house peak simply watching everything all around. Two mockingbirds were clearly not happy with the buzzard's presence in their neighborhood. They kept buzzing around and dive-bombing at him, but he ignored them for the most part. They were still shrilling and buzzing around him as I left them behind. A couple blocks later a young man walking his big black dog passed me. We chatted for a moment, and he told me he took his dog for a three and a half mile walk every morning. I commented that was great for both of them, and he grinned as he replied: "I don't know if I do it more for him or me." They're not the only ones. I usually see quite a few people walking their dogs every morning.

In addition to the wild and domestic life along the way, I'm always interested in the plants and landscaping of the various homes I pass. I enjoy seeing all the different ways people use to beautify their homes and yards. As I walk I also enjoy the sun's warming rays and the balmy breeze that kisses my cheeks.

In the winter I wear gloves and a fleece-lined jacket, and my breath is steamy in the cold air as I take my brisk morning walk. Whatever the season, it's always a joy to spend this time outdoors. There is something about experiencing nature directly that is exhilarating for body, mind and spirit.

By contrast, I also enjoy my indoor workouts at the YMCA. At the moment I'm working out with a trainer twice a week and also taking a Pilates class once or twice a week. Learning new routines and stretching muscles, tendons and joints in new ways is a challenge, especially for an old man! Yet, it's also fun to work with expert instructors who know just how much to "push" their students, and do it in such a caring way. I know they want to help me succeed in reaching my modest goals.

Tennis is another physical activity that I thoroughly enjoy. I play in the Senior Men's group at the "Y" about twice a week, and I'm far from one of the best players. Still, I get into the "zone" at my level of play, focus totally on the game, and lose all sense of concern about anything outside the tennis court. Win or lose, the camaraderie is always great, and the two or three hours spent in the sunshine is wonderful. It's also a great way to get my vitamin D!

A final activity that gives me great pleasure is working in our yard for three or four hours most weekends. I enjoy planting, transplanting, watering and weeding in our small box gardens in the backyard, and I even enjoy spending an hour or so weeding out the ever-recurring crabgrass from our lawn.

The rewards are immense. In addition to the quiet inner joy that I feel as I'm puttering around the yard, we enjoy the Swiss chard, sweet basil, tomatoes, chives and other produce that we harvest from our little box gardens a couple times a week. Their freshness as part of our lunch or supper is marvelous. Then there is the indefinable joy of sitting on our back patio in the evening, drinking in the simple beauty of the flowers in our yard, the butterflies flitting around them, and the birds at play in the birdbath.

Exercise is whatever you make of it. A lot depends on the mental attitude you have about it. It can be dull and boring if that's what you make of it, or it can be full of life-giving energy and joy if that's what you make of it. Here are key pointers that help make it enjoyable as a lifetime kind of activity: Put variety into your exercise program; make it companionable by doing it with others when you can; and make it something you enjoy doing. None of this is automatic. The more energy you put into making your exercise program something that you enjoy doing, the more it will reward you!

Reminders

1. Exercise for at least 45 minutes six days a week.

2. Simple walking provides wonderful health benefits.

3. A simple pedometer is a very useful exercise tool.

4. Physical fitness is essential to overall health, but it is not a health panacea by itself.

5. Variety adds interest to any exercise program.

6. Companionship in exercise is a good way to boost your enjoyment.

7. Above all, learn to invest joy into your exercise program.

CHAPTER ELEVEN

Personal and Mental Hygiene

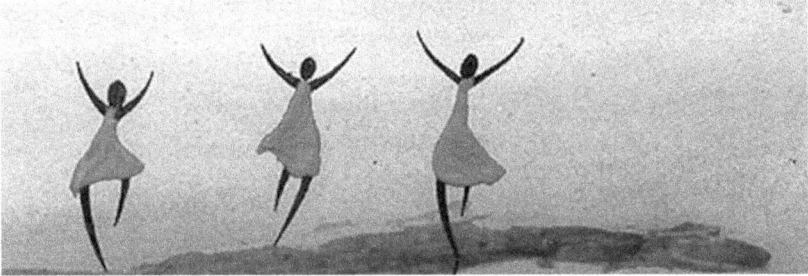

Adam learns that hygiene has a deeper, broader impact on health than most people realize. It's one of the basic pillars that supports lifelong health. This chapter focuses on personal and mental hygiene because this is where people can take effective actions to protect their health. Adam knows some of this, but some of it is eye-opening.

Hygiene

The word hygiene comes from Hygeia, the Greek goddess of health. It was said that she prevented sickness and preserved health, so her name is associated with health and cleanliness. Today, hygiene is defined as a set of practices performed for the preservation of health, or the science that deals with the promotion and preservation of health.

The Sanitation Movement of the 1800s deserves credit for major advances in public health. Its emphasis was on cleaning up urban wastes and providing clean public water supplies. We now take an abundant supply of clean water for granted, but there are many places in the world where clean water is scarce. Growing up in Africa, and later working in areas where the water supply was limited at times, I learned to appreciate the blessings of clean water fairly early in life.

Bathing or showering on a regular basis is clearly a good idea, even though little boys (and sometimes bigger ones) may occasionally resist. In chapter one, I described the "overhead bucket" arrangement we had for bathing when we lived in the Dembos area of Angola. That innovative idea always made the bath interesting!

Later, when we lived in Gondar, Ethiopia, the city water system shut down frequently during the latter part of the dry season. Sometimes we only had water coming into our home for an hour or so in the middle of the night. We had a large metal tank as a back-up reservoir, but even that went dry on occasion. We became expert at a primitive kind of water recycling. We used our dirty dish and bath water to flush the toilet to avoid using up precious clean water.

These experiences made me realize what a luxury it is to have abundant clean water. When I saw women in rural areas carry large jugs of water for long distances for all their household needs, I knew their water was a precious commodity. It supplied their drinking, cooking and washing needs for the day, so it was used very frugally. Unfortunately, it often came from unsafe sources. It's not surprising that contagious illnesses were major problems.

Research studies reveal that simple, consistent hand washing remains one of the best ways to prevent the spread of many common infections. Viral diseases such as the common cold are frequently spread by hand-to-hand contact. Yet, even in places with excellent public water supplies and clean facilities, handwashing is often neglected. It's a good habit to wash one's hands often enough to keep them clean, particularly after using the bathroom, working in dirty environments and before eating meals. Handwashing is also a good idea after visiting hospitals or after shaking a lot of hands.

Dental Hygiene

Dental hygiene is more important than many people realize. I learned this the hard way. Even though my parents often told me to brush my teeth after meals, I was not good about this. As a result, I developed many cavities in my teeth as I was growing up. Then, at age 20, when I was in college, I suffered from a serious abscess at the root of one of my upper front teeth that gave me a terrible toothache. When the dentist examined me, he shook his head and told me there was nothing he could do except pull out the offending tooth and put me on an antibiotic.

After the infection subsided, he fit me with a partial denture that I had to take out and clean every night. I was literally forced into better dental hygiene by this process. A few years later, I had the partial denture replaced by a "permanent" bridge. It served me well for over 30 years, but then it too had to be replaced at a cost of several thousand dollars. All told, I've spent many thousands of dollars on my teeth because of early poor dental hygiene.

According to CDC statistics, almost a fourth of all adults who reach the age of 65 in the United States are edentulous, meaning they have lost all their teeth. Any inconvenience or discomfort of wearing dentures that may not fit well is compounded by the inability to chew food well and the loss of enjoying many foods previously liked. Edentulous elderly people tend to eat soft foods that don't require much chewing, but are not nutrient-rich. A downward health spiral may occur as poor nutrition leads to poor immune status and increased risk of many illnesses.

I am fortunate. I have a mouth full of assorted fillings and a permanent bridge, but otherwise my teeth are in better shape now than they were at age 20. I use "Go Betweens" to clean out any food debris between my teeth that a regular toothbrush can't reach. I brush my teeth carefully three times a day, and I floss them every evening after my last meal. When I see her, my dental hygienist compliments me on the good condition of my teeth and gums. More importantly, I enjoy eating good food more than ever.

Is it smart to take good care of your teeth?

- To avoid the pain of severe toothaches?

- To avoid the cost of extensive dental work?

- To enjoy good food all your life?

Nearly everyone would say "Yes" to these questions. Yet many fail Dental Care 101. Perhaps the true nitty-gritty question is: Are you willing to devote the time and effort to brush your teeth faithfully after every meal? It's a simple enough habit, but it took me a long time to learn its great value.

Kitchen Hygiene

Hygiene is especially important in the kitchen because food contamination is a cause of preventable illness. Beyond the need to routinely wash hands and utensils, there are several points worth emphasizing.

Whoever does food preparation should be free of contagious disease. If a person preparing food has a cold and is coughing, sneezing and nose-blowing a lot, someone else should take over in the kitchen if possible. The same principle applies if the food handler has open sores of the hands. These are simple common-sense rules. Nobody wants to eat food handled by someone who is shedding contagious germs.

Most contaminated food outbreaks today are due to contamination before the food is ever bought at the marketplace. The most commonly contaminated foods are fresh produce and meats. The source of contamination can go as far back as the fields where the produce is grown. In the case of meat, contamination often occurs at the slaughterhouse. In either case, it is important for these foods to be handled and washed especially carefully in the home kitchen.

Even when packaged produce is labeled as having been "Triple-Washed," it's important to wash it again at home. Testing of such produce shows that it can still carry some germs. Except for fruits and vegetables that can be peeled, we wash all fresh vegetables and fruit in a colander before eating or cooking them.

Meat is more complicated. Testing shows that much of the meat sold in supermarkets is contaminated with bacteria and traces of feces coming from the animals themselves in the slaughtering process. Since meat is usually grilled, fried or roasted long enough to kill all bacteria, it usually does not cause a problem when it's eaten. The problem comes in handling it before it's cooked. Utensils, cutting-boards and plates that hold uncooked meat often test positive for bacteria afterwards. The same is true for the hands of the cook.

What this means is that meat must always be handled super-carefully. When cutting-boards, plates and knives are used with raw meat, always wash them immediately after use. Never use a cutting-board for other foods after it has been used for meat. Likewise, anyone who handles meat while it is raw needs to wash his or her hands before going on to work with other foods.

A final kitchen note: Any leftovers after a meal need to be refrigerated promptly. Food left to sit around for a couple hours at room temperature can become a source of food poisoning, simply because a few bacteria can multiply rapidly to thousands or millions in a short time. That's all it takes to cause food-borne illness the next time it's eaten.

Smoking and Hygiene

Smoking is poor hygiene. Smokers' lungs become dirty gray in color compared to the pink color of healthy lungs, making it obvious that smoking is a non-hygienic practice. Unfortunately, the impact of smoking is broader than causing the lungs of smokers to develop a dirty gray color. It's not only poor personal hygiene; it's also poor community hygiene.

Tobacco products designed for human use cause serious internal chemical pollution. Over 7,000 chemicals are released and inhaled while a cigarette is burning; 250 of these are known to be harmful to health. At least 69 can cause cancer. Smoking causes cancers of the lung, esophagus, larynx, mouth, throat, kidney, bladder, pancreas, stomach, and cervix, as well as acute myeloid leukemia.

Smoking is also a major contributor to heart disease, stroke, and chronic lung disease. It's the leading cause of premature, preventable death in the United States and around the world. Every year, over 400,000 premature deaths occur due to smoking in the USA. Worldwide, it causes over five million deaths annually.

All forms of tobacco are polluting. Smoking tobacco, chewing tobacco or using snuff are all hazardous to health. There is simply no way of using tobacco that is not internally polluting. Secondhand smoke can also affect the health of non-smokers when they are around smokers. It is a cause of cancer, heart disease, and respiratory disease. In the United States, about 50,000 non-smokers die annually because of inhaling secondhand smoke.

The nicotine in tobacco is what makes it so addicting. Nicotine is a potent chemical that stimulates the brain and nervous system. Paradoxically, it also has a calming effect. Within seconds of inhaling, nicotine hits the brain with instant effects. That's what makes it so enticing. Unfortunately, the smoking "package" that carries the nicotine has the serious long-term consequences that we've discussed.

Nicotine patches applied to the skin have helped many people withdraw from their tobacco addiction. Nicotine gum and electronic cigarettes are other devices invented to deliver nicotine without tobacco. These are useful, but with prolonged use, long-term addiction to nicotine remains a concern. The best practice is to avoid addiction by never using any tobacco product in the first place.

Marijuana

Marijuana is another plant that has potent effects on the body when it is smoked. A study reported in the *Journal of the American Medical Association* (JAMA) concluded that occasional marijuana use over a 20 year period did not seem to damage lung function, but heavy use did have damaging effects.[20]

This does not mean that light use of marijuana is harmless. Marijuana can cause acute psychic disturbances, and long-term mental health problems such as depression and increased risks of suicide are a concern. A recently published study of marijuana use in teenagers who were tracked over 25 years showed a significant loss of intellectual ability and drop in IQ by age 38. The loss of intellectual function was not fully restored by stopping marijuana as adults.[21]

Marijuana can be used for the relief of several medical problems. The issue of medical marijuana has been controversial, but its use for medical reasons is increasingly recognized as valid. Twenty states have passed laws to legalize medical marijuana. New Hampshire passed a law to legalize it medically in July, 2013. Illinois became the twentieth state to do this in August, 2013. On August 29th, 2013, the U.S. Department of Justice announced it would not challenge state marijuana laws.[22]

Although there are valid reasons for the medical use of marijuana, its use by healthy people is not a good idea. As with tobacco, it's smart to never begin using marijuana in the first place.

---

20. M.J. Pletcher, MD, MPH et al. "Association between Marijuana Exposure and Pulmonary Function Over 20 Years," *Journal of the American Medical Association*, Vol 307, No. 2, January 11, 2012; pp 173-180.

21. http://www.medicinenet.com/marijuana/article.htm

22. http://medicalmarijuana.procon.org/view.timeline.php?timelineID=000026

Prescription and OTC Drugs

Medications are a health hazard that few people think about. Yet, most medications are chemicals that affect the body. Most of them have toxic effects on the body. The research done by pharmaceutical companies on new drugs is designed to find dose levels that are effective and relatively free of dangerous side effects.

However, all drugs have potentially dangerous effects, and in some cases the line between an effective and a toxic dose is a fine line. Other factors can make this hazard more treacherous. Age makes a difference in how well a drug is tolerated, simply because of age-related processing differences. The young and the old are especially vulnerable to these problems.

Regardless of age, individuals can vary widely in the way their bodies handle or process different drugs. This variability makes it difficult to predict how any individual may react to new medications. In prescribing dosages of medications new to any patient, the advice to "start low and go slow" is wise, even with well-known drugs.

When a person is on more than one medication, drug interactions become an increasing problem. The risk of potentially dangerous interactions rises rapidly with the number of medications being taken, including over-the-counter medications. Since millions of patients are on many medications, this is not a small problem. Almost half of all Americans are on at least one prescription drug, and many older Americans are on multiple medications. Medication side effects have been one of the leading causes of hospitalization and death in the United States for many years.

Over-the-counter (OTC) drugs can also cause problems. Many people think OTC drugs are perfectly safe, but no drug is totally safe. All drugs can affect bodily functions in profound ways, and some of these ways are damaging to health. This is true for every kind of drug, legal or illegal. Never take any drug without good reason. When medications are needed to support health, they should be taken appropriately.

Many health problems can be prevented with healthy lifestyles, minimizing or avoiding any need for medications. Most people like the idea of good health free of the risks (and costs) of medications. Lifestyle changes can offer this option, sometimes restoring health to the point that no medications are needed. Most physicians can help patients make positive lifestyle changes, providing good support for patients who are motivated to improve their health through a healthier lifestyle.

If it's possible to come off any medication, this should be done under a physician's supervision. It can take time to adjust to the withdrawal of a drug. One's physician knows best how to synchronize any withdrawal and adjustment processes.

Mental Hygiene

I joined the United States Public Health Service in 1964, fresh out of internship and a year of residency. I requested assignment to the Indian Health Service, thinking I could do some good and get some valuable experience during my two years of service to our country. My hopes were dashed when I received my assignment papers. I was assigned to the Bureau of Prisons for two years. Specifically, I was commissioned as a Medical Officer at the Federal Reformatory in Chillicothe, Ohio.

The reformatory had about 1300 young men, a majority of whom were in their late teens or early twenties. Most came out of seriously dysfunctional backgrounds. Many came with psychopathic or sociopathic problems of varying severity. Putting them all together in a confined institution created a social situation that was like a simmering cauldron underneath a tenuous outward calm imposed by the security system.

We had a psychiatric consultant who came to the reformatory twice a week. He did a little psychotherapy, but his time was taken up mainly with diagnostic classification of new inmates and associated paperwork. Most of the inmates had fairly good health physically, but their mental/emotional health was not so good. I learned a lot about psychopathology during my two-year tour of duty.

We had a daily "sick call" clinic every morning for inmates who had any kind of health complaint. Most complaints had to do with minor colds or ailments, though occasionally someone came through with an illness requiring more attention. We had a small 15-bed in-patient facility where we could observe or care for sicker inmates. I learned very quickly that getting admitted to our facility was prized so much that some inmates would feign symptoms of any illness they thought might get them admitted. I found that I had to make decisions based on my physical exam or basic lab tests, not on presenting symptoms. This was true for out-patients also, as inmates tried to get "Medical Releases" to get out of work details.

Although they were self-centered, most inmates were angry with the world and themselves. They had low self-regard. The most common reason for me to be called back to the reformatory at night was to treat an inmate who had lacerated his wrist or arm. After caring for the laceration, the inmate was taken back to his cell, or occasionally moved to an isolation cell. Sometimes I was called back an hour or so later because the same inmate had ripped out his sutures with his teeth.

The reformatory environment did not enhance good mental health, regardless of the sincerity of "reform-minded" planners. The concentration of psychopathology in the institution was simply too overwhelming for effective reform for most inmates.

Unfortunately, while psychopathology is not so concentrated in most places outside of prisons, mental health is also a problem in the world at large. Time-pressure problems, stressful conditions, emotional conflicts and physical ailments are all factors.

Anger, Depression, and Loneliness

Anger and depression are clearly not healthy for us in the long run. When a person is angry, he secretes high levels of cortisol, the "fight or flight" hormone. In situations of acute danger, that's necessary, because cortisol tones the body up for fight or flight, but it's not good when the cortisol levels remain high due to chronic stress. Persistently high levels depress the immune system, raise blood pressure, and increase the risk of diabetes.

Depression is more common today than it was 50 years ago, despite rising standards of living. Yet, rates of depression have climbed every decade in the USA over the last 50 years. Twenty million Americans suffer from depression today. We don't know why it has become an epidemic. Economic self-sufficiency is helpful, but wealth clearly does not insulate people from depression.

When I was teaching at the Public Health College in Gondar, Ethiopia from 1967-69, one of my classes did an informal household survey of mental well-being of villagers in a roadside town of about 2000 people. It turned out that statistics were similar to statistics in the United States in the 1960s, even though the USA had far greater economic wealth. Most rural villagers in Ethiopia at that time earned less than $1 a day.

International surveys confirm that mental well-being is not well correlated with economic wealth. An article by Matt Haikin in May, 2012 reveals statistics that support a thesis that the poor in low-income countries are better-off in terms of mental health than the poor in high-income countries. Overall, the USA had a much higher prevalence of mental illness than many low and middle-income countries.[23]

Whatever the reasons, depression is often associated with feelings of disconnection. According to Abraham Maslow and Heinz Kohut, leaders

---

23. http://www.hiidunia.com/wp-content/uploads/downloads/2013/03/Poverty-Well-being-PUBLISHED.pdf

in psychology and psychiatry in the mid-twentieth century, the need for human connection is very basic. They theorized that a lack of "belonging-ness" was a major cause of mental health problems.[24]

We have more drugs to treat depression and other mental health prob-lems than we have ever had before. Prescribed in record amounts, they may help control various mental health symptoms, but they are not a panacea. Robert Whitaker, in his award-winning book, *Anatomy of an Epidemic*, lays out evidence that the medications used to treat this growing epidemic of mental disorders may actually have become part of the problem.[25]

Several leading psychologists and psychiatrists agree that drugs are not the best way to treat depression. Dr. Martin Seligman, author of *Flourish*, and head of the Department of Psychology at the University of Pennsylvania, provides evidence that treating depression through positive psychology is more effective than treating with medications.[26]

Dr. James Gordon, Founder and Director of the Center for Mind-Body Medicine at Georgetown Medical School and author of the book *Unstuck*, suffered from depression as a young adult. Saying that depression is not an end point, but a sign of being out of balance, he advises making life changes to help restore balance. He describes seven stages of getting "unstuck" from depression, and has taught this method effectively for many years.[27]

Sunlight has been known to boost mood for many years. It seems to activate brain neurons that raise serotonin levels and this in turn is cor-related with improvements in mood. Vitamin D, the sunshine vitamin, is also gaining credit as a possible factor in improving mental health. On the

24. Kristin Neff. *Self-Compassion*, (New York, NY: HarperCollins, 2011), p. 64.

25. http://www.madinamerica.com/madinamerica.com/
Whitakerblog/29EF57FB-66DC-41F4-9E57-ACC6E237A981.html

26. http://www.authentichappiness.sas.upenn.edu/Default.aspx

27. http://cmbm.org/about/james-s-gordon-md-founder-director/

other hand, the absence of sunlight for long periods of time is associated with Seasonal Affective Disorder (SAD,) a seasonal type of depression.

Regular exercise has been shown in many studies to be effective in preventing and/or treating depression. Dr Henry Lodge, co-author of *Younger Next Year,* provides solid reasons as to why this is true. Exercise promotes the formation and release of abundant natural chemicals in the body that stimulate growth of healthy new cells throughout the body, including the brain. When regular exercise is combined with companionship and caring connections with others, the therapeutic effect is powerful. Brain imaging today literally lets us see this kind of positive impact in the brain.

What this suggests is that getting regular exercise outdoors in the sunlight may provide a triple-barreled boost to mental health. Exercise itself has proven to be valuable for mental health. Much evidence suggests that sunlight and vitamin D are also good for mental health. The combination of all three may be more effective than medications!

Nourish the Mind!

Isaac Ray, a founder of the American Psychiatric Association, defined mental hygiene as the "art of preserving the mind against influences that inhibit its energy, quality, or development." The World Health Organization defines mental health as "a state of well-being in which the individual realizes his or her own abilities, can cope with the normal stresses of life, can work productively and fruitfully, and is able to make a contribution to his or her community."[28]

Regardless of how it is phrased, the idea of nourishing our minds is worthwhile. Mental health statistics show only 20 percent of the adult population flourishing with the healthiest psychosocial functioning. Much in our world culture today detracts from good mental health. Shielding our

---

28. https://en.wikipedia.org/wiki/Mental_health

minds from negative influences while promoting positive ones is an age-old endeavor. No matter how this concept is framed, it always remains relevant.

Perhaps Paul put it best in his advice to the people of Philippi two thousand years ago. "Fix your thoughts on what is true and good and right. Think about things that are pure and lovely, and dwell on the fine, good things in others. Think about all you can praise God for and be glad about... and the God of peace will be with you." I can't say it better.

Major hygienic emphases to remember:

- Washing hands regularly is the best way to prevent spread of infectious diseases.

- Dental hygiene is important for general health as well as oral health.

- Minimize medication use as much as possible (with physician help.)

- Don't smoke or use tobacco products.

- Foster positive mental influences and avoid negative ones as much as possible.

CHAPTER TWELVE

Good Environmental Hygiene

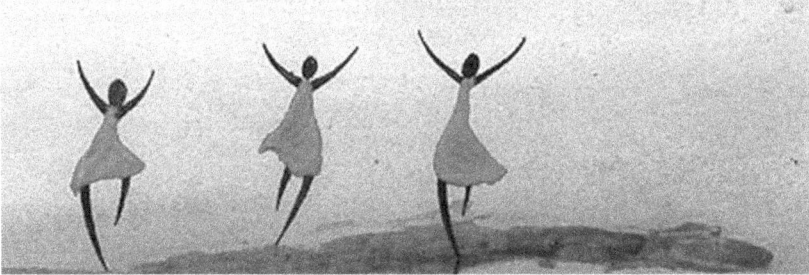

Environmental hygiene is something that most people agree on in principle. After all, who doesn't want clean safe surroundings? The difficulty (or the devil) is in the details. It is often complicated and costly to put good environmental practices into effect, and because of this, shortcuts can be very tempting. Here, Adam gets a better picture of the challenges involved, but also gains a better understanding of what committed individuals can do to safeguard their own health.

Environmental Hygiene

The environment we live in is important to our health. Hippocrates realized this 2600 years ago. He challenged the thinking of his day with his teaching about the environment, summarizing this in his masterful treatise on *Air, Water, and Places*. Before then, health was thought to be dependent on the whims of the gods, but Hippocrates showed that environmental influences had an important impact on health.

We began to gain greater scientific understanding about this after a cholera epidemic swept through London in 1854. The English physician John Snow studied its distribution and concluded that contaminated water from the Broad Street well was a factor in spreading the disease.[29] The microbial theory of contagion was not yet accepted, but Snow's work made an impact. He is called the Father of Epidemiology because of his analysis of the problem.

His work was a key influence in the Sanitary Movement of the next hundred years. That movement did much to clean up unsanitary conditions in towns and cities around the world, but water and sanitation challenges still need our attention today. The book, *Water and Sanitation-Related Diseases and the Environment*, edited by Janine M. H. Selendy and published by Wiley-Blackwell in 2011, goes into today's water and sanitation problems in some depth. I contributed the chapter on the Zimbabwe cholera epidemic of 2008-09. Many other current environmental health problems are addressed by other authors.

Malaria

Malaria is a complicated disease that is a major problem around the world, especially in Africa. In 1939, my father came close to dying from blackwater fever, a dreaded complication of malaria that still has a high fatality rate today. I had malaria as a child growing up in Angola, so I have a personal interest in it. Unhappily, millions of adults and children still contract malaria today, and it's still a major cause of death in the tropical world.

People catch malaria when bitten by mosquitoes that carry the malaria parasites from those who are infected. The World Health Organization (WHO) developed Integrated Vector Management (IVM) as its newest strategy to prevent and control malaria. Anopheles mosquitoes are the vector (carrier) that must be controlled to stop the spread of the disease, so a big part of this effort is a multi-pronged strategy to control this mosquito.

A detailed discussion of this strategy is beyond the scope of this book,

29. http://en.wikipedia.org/wiki/John_Snow

but measures include environmental management as well as biological and chemical methods of fighting against infected mosquitoes. In terms of personal prevention, the main options today are the use of insecticide-treated mosquito nets, taking some form of medication to prevent malaria, or moving out of malarious areas. Treated mosquito nets are effective if used.

Pesticides as an Environmental Health Hazard

New environmental health problems began to be recognized in the United States in mid-twentieth century, and many of them remain major challenges today. Rachel Carson, a biologist with the Fish and Wildlife Service, began to study the effects of pesticides on the environment in the 1950s.

After her research showed the devastating effect of pesticides on birds and other wildlife, Carson wrote the book, *Silent Spring*. Its publication in 1962 sparked the modern environmental movement, leading to the formation of the Environmental Protection Agency (EPA) in 1970. Ironically, overall pesticide use in the USA has more than doubled since *Silent Spring*, but that does not lessen the impact of Carson's achievements.[30]

Carson alerted us to the hazards of pesticides. Since then, some like DDT and chlordane have been banned or phased out, but many are still in use. Residues of banned pesticides can persist for decades. Doris Rapp, MD, author of the book, *Our Toxic World: A Wake-up Call*, explained some of these residual effects in an interview reported on the internet. She also notes that children are much more sensitive than adults to the toxic effects of chemicals, with safe levels for children being at least ten times lower than

---

30. http://en.wikipedia.org/wiki/Rachel_Carson

for adults.[31] The Environmental Working Group (EWG) publishes a helpful list: EWG Shopper's Guide to Pesticides in Produce™ that is free. It lists the most heavily contaminated "Dirty Dozen" foods, as well as the "Clean 15" that are low in pesticides. The Dirty Dozen foods include peaches, apples, bell peppers, celery, cherries, nectarines, strawberries, kale, lettuce, imported grapes, carrots, and pears. Organically grown produce is the safest source of these foods. If you can't get organic foods, buy the conventional kind, but wash or peel them thoroughly.

The Clean 15 include onions, avocado, sweet corn, pineapple, mango, asparagus, sweet peas, kiwi, cabbage, eggplant, papaya, watermelon, broccoli, and sweet potatoes. Their contamination is so minor that it is OK to buy them from conventional sources. The EWG Shopper's Guide is updated every year, so it's best to check it online at least annually.[32]

The danger of pesticides was dramatized by the tragic death of 23 school children in India after eating a free school lunch in July, 2013. It was thought that the cooking oil used for the meal had been stored in a used container of the toxic pesticide, monochrotophos. Most countries around the world have banned this pesticide because of its toxicity, but Indian authorities claim it's safe if used as directed. The problem, obviously, is that it's deadly if there is a slip-up.[33]

Other Community Influences on Health

The communities we live in have more influence on health than many people realize. Communities with good sidewalks and nice parks make it

31. http://www.sixwise.com/newsletters/05/10/12/why-banned-toxic-substances-diazinon--amp-dursban-are-still-in-use-today-an-interview-with-environ.htm

32. http://www.ewg.org/foodnews/summary.php

33. http://indiatoday.intoday.in/story/bihar-mid-day-meal-tragedy-cheap-food-vs-death-by-poisoning/1/296790.html

attractive for people to get out and walk. Good bike paths and trails encourage bicycling. Positive environmental features like these help promote active exercise.

Local farmer's markets makes it easier for people to get fresh produce. Community Supported Agriculture (CSA) is a good way for farmers and consumers to share risks and rewards by pooling their resources and crops. In return for buying a share of the crop in advance, consumers get boxes or baskets of produce every week during the growing season. They benefit from eating truly fresh produce, much of it organically grown.

On the other hand, negative community factors exist that make it difficult for many people to adopt healthy lifestyles. Urban centers may lack any good nutritional or recreational sites. Industrial air pollution, afflicting many cities, has a negative environmental impact on health, especially for children. Rates of asthma and respiratory infection are worse in such areas. Air pollution is also associated with increased risks of cancer, chronic lung disease, and chronic heart disease.

Industrial financial interests often make the bottom line more important than community health. Short-term profit may trump long-term safety and environmental concerns, with the result that health-endangering business practices may prevail. When true, this can make it much harder than it should be for individuals to follow a healthy lifestyle. (See Appendix A to review other health issues related to business factors beyond individual control.)

Excess Radiation

Radiation hazards are another environmental concern. Everyone receives a little natural background radiation every day. This comes from the natural radioactivity of the earth as well as cosmic radiation from space. Some people get more of this than others. For example, airline crews that spend hundreds of hours in flight every year get more cosmic radiation than most earthbound people, but health risks due to this are minimal.

People who work in certain industries have occupational exposure to radiation. Where the risk is significant, workers wear monitoring badges to make sure they do not receive unsafe levels of radiation. Most of us do not need such badges, but we are exposed to medical radiation from x-rays and CT scans. Today, safeguards are in place to keep diagnostic medical radiation at low levels, but that should not make anyone complacent about x-ray's dangers.

X-rays were discovered in 1895. Early workers in this field suffered serious radiation burns before we learned about its dangers. Thomas Edison's young assistant, Clarence Daily, worked extensively with x-rays, and was so "poisonously affected" by them that his hair fell out and his scalp became ulcerated. Later, he developed severe cancerous ulcerations of his hands and arms, to the point of requiring amputation of both arms. In spite of the surgery, radiation induced cancer caused his death in 1904 at age 39. His death led to the development of many of the radiation safeguards we use today.[34]

X-rays cause damage by ripping electrons off cells, breaking chemical bonds, and creating unstable molecules called free radicals. They can also cause mutations and other genetic damage. Some of this damage can be repaired by the body, but much of it is cumulative. The risk from a few x-rays is negligible, but the risk of cancer from numerous x-rays over many years is a concern, especially if relatively high doses are involved.[35]

Rapidly growing cells are especially sensitive to the damaging effects of radiation. Small children have greater risk of damage from x-rays than adults because of this. They also have more risk of delayed damage, such as cancer

34. http://www.e-radiography.net/articles/biologicaleffects.htm

35. http://www.physics.isu.edu/radinf/risk.htm

showing up years later, simply because they have a longer expected lifespan than adults. Embryos and fetuses are the most sensitive of all to radiation damage. That's why pregnant women are discouraged from getting x-rays unless absolutely necessary.

To summarize, medical x-rays are useful diagnostic tools, but they should be used only when the information they provide is important for diagnostic or clinical management purposes. Their use is more controversial when they are used for broad screening programs such as mammograms, where the risk to benefit ratio is debated. As with medications, x-rays should not be used without clear reasons for their use.

Problems with BPA (Bisphenol A)

Research at Harvard's School of Public Health recently found that the chemical BPA, often used in the lining of food and beverage cans, is released into food and absorbed by humans in much higher amounts than previously known. Volunteers who had one serving of canned soup daily for five days were found to have concentrations of BPA in their urine more than one thousand times greater than from one serving of freshly made soup every day for five days.[36]

Invented by a Russian scientist in 1891, BPA has been in commercial use for over 50 years. Eight billion pounds are used by manufacturers annually to line metal cans, make plastic containers and bottles, and other uses. Since BPA is an endocrine disrupter, there is concern about its impact on the reproductive process. Many countries have banned its use for infant products, and infant bottles and pacifiers that are BPA-free are now marketed in the USA.[37]

Early BPA studies showed interference with reproduction in animals.

36. http://www.hsph.harvard.edu/news/press-releases/canned-soup-bpa/

37. http://en.wikipedia.org/wiki/Bisphenol_A

BPA has also been linked with diabetes, heart disease, and other disorders in humans. The new Harvard study is the first one to show such high levels coming from eating standard canned foods. The food industry denies any danger to humans from the use of BPA, but the Harvard study will stimulate further research. The Food and Drug Administration currently has the BPA problem under study.[38]

This BPA report highlights several issues we've reviewed about chemicals in our lives. It reveals the typical industry reaction of denial when health concerns are raised. It shows how long it can take to verify concerns about chemicals already in use. It reveals the difficulty of convincing industry and regulatory agencies to make real change. Finally, it shows why the Precautionary Principle (which I discuss more fully in Appendix A) is needed. Chemicals like BPA should not be used in connection with food until proven safe.

The food industry has begun to use BPA-free plastics for infant bottles and some kinds of water bottles. Eventually, it will probably use BPA-free metal cans. Until then, be cautious about using canned foods.

Waste Disposal

Waste collection and disposal presents another environmental challenge. Every American throws out nearly one and a half tons of solid waste every year, for a national total of over 400 million tons of trash a year. Most of this goes to landfills, which takes trash out of sight for most of us. Unfortunately, it also takes it out of mind for many of us. In spite of careful management of landfills today, there are major long-range concerns about waste management and landfills today.

Three specific stories about waste management are instructive. The first illustrates how the issue of waste management can become complicated,

---

38. http://www.niehs.nih.gov/health/topics/agents/sya-bpa/

even when a technical solution is fairly straightforward. The Grand Canyon National Park planned to ban disposable plastic water bottles in the park effective January 1, 2012 because they were a major source of trash. The plan was modeled after a successful ban of plastic water bottles by Zion National Park in 2008 that won high praise and awards.

The Grand Canyon plan was approved by all superiors up the line in the National Park Service. It took most of a year to get ready for the ban. The park installed multiple water filling stations around the park for reusable bottles, so access to good drinking water would not be a problem. Less than a month before the ban was set to begin, officials at the Grand Canyon Park were told the ban was being tabled by the head of the National Park Service in Washington.

The officially cited reason for tabling the ban was a need to better study its impact, but this came up only after the ban was questioned by Coca-Cola® shortly before it was to begin. Coca-Cola® is a distributor of water under the Dasani® brand. It is also a major donor to the National Park Foundation. Mr. Stephan Martin, top park official at the Grand Canyon was disturbed by the decision, saying "the idea of being influenced unduly by business" was an ethical issue.[39]

After an avalanche of protests when the news about tabling the ban was publicized, the National Park Service reversed itself and re-instituted the ban. Apparently it was responding to expressed public unhappiness. In any case, the ban was activated in February, 2012. By all accounts, it has been successful in terms of improved waste management and decreased littering of disposable water bottles.

Stories from Earth University

---

39. http://www.nytimes.com/2011/11/10/science/earth/parks-chief-blocked-plan-for-grand-canyon-bottle-ban.html

Earth University in Costa Rica was established in 1986 with the specific goal of preparing young people from Latin America and other developing areas to contribute to sustainable development of their home countries. Its four-year undergraduate program in agricultural sciences and natural resources management provides a world class scientific and technological education that emphasizes ethical values combined with environmental and social commitment.[40]

An August, 2013 news release from Earth University tells two stories of "Converting Waste into Opportunity." The first story is about Monica Lozano, an Earth University alumna from Colombia who learned that waste can be converted into useful material. Since returning to Colombia she has had a major impact on the field of waste management there. She worked for the government for a time, where she played a role as Coordinator of the Clean Agricultural Program, including the creation of Colombia's first organic food certification.

She then moved into the private sector as an independent agricultural consultant before she went on to establish her own business, entitled Sea Soil. Today she leads a project involving three companies that work to improve waste management practices throughout the city of Bogota with its 7.5 million inhabitants. The project collects organic waste and composts it into a product that can be put back into local crops. It provides environmental education as it does this, and has impacted thousands of lives.

Monica has demonstrated that sustainable practices can protect natural resources while generating a profit for the companies involved. She credits Earth University for her success, saying it taught her "sustainability in all its splendor."

The second story is about Rui Leonardo Madime of the class of 2013. Coming from Mozambique, he became interested in bio-digester technol-

---

40. http://www.earth.ac.cr/about-earth/earth-facts/

ogy at Earth University. This became the focus of his studies and research. In his third year, he did his internship in the Yucatan region of Mexico. During his fifteen weeks there, he taught the community about bio-digesters that convert animal excrement into fire, and he became known as "the man with new fire."

Working with an agro-ecological school there, he found families that were willing to install the new bio-digester systems. Incredibly, in his short time there, he persuaded 46 families to adopt these new systems which they could use as a source of usable energy. He was so successful in this cross-cultural venture that the W. K. Kellogg Foundation is financing the installation of one thousand additional systems in the area. "The man with new fire" will take his technology skills and his passion back to his homeland to help his communities there make the kinds of changes that will help them deal with wastes in a productive way.

These stories let us know that great as the environmental challenges are that confront all of us, we should never throw our hands up in despair. Sustainable solutions can be found and applied!

The Campaign for Safe Cosmetics

Individuals and corporations can work together to improve corporate products for the benefit of the entire community. A good example of this can be seen in the Campaign for Safe Cosmetics, an initiative that began in 2004. Nonprofit organizations teamed up with firms in the cosmetics industry to cooperatively search for solutions to making and marketing safe cosmetic and personal care products. Over 1500 companies signed the compact to work on this problem.

A news release on November 30, 2011 announced that 321 firms had met the goals of the compact, and another 111 firms had made good progress towards these goals. "These companies have truly broken the mold," said

Janet Nudelman, program director of the Breast Cancer Fund, a founding member of the Campaign for Safe Cosmetics. "They are leading the cosmetics industry toward safety, showing it's possible to make products with full transparency and without using hazardous chemicals."[41]

Conclusion

This completes our survey of major environmental health issues. It does not cover all of them by any means, but it highlights our most common concerns. Many environmental issues are complicated, affecting nearly every aspect of our lives. Unsafe environmental practices can have negative impacts on nutritional fitness, physical fitness and mental/emotional fitness. The web of life is exceedingly intricate, and ramifications of unsafe environmental practices are far-reaching.

There are no easy answers for resolving many of these issues, but we must keep doing our best. There is satisfaction to be found in doing our best for our families, our communities, and our planet. In spite of corporate influences that can make healthy lifestyles hard to attain, the individual pursuit of healthy ways of living is valuable. If corporations can be involved in designing true win/win solutions to environmental problems, as in the campaign for safe cosmetics, all the better. The more we do this, the more hope we can have for our future. That's why healthy living is the core message of this book.

A Few Practical Tips:

- Plant a small organic garden at home to enjoy the freshest healthy veggies. The garden doesn't have to be large to be helpful. We have a small backyard in San Antonio, but the terrain where we live is very rocky. Our solution was to put in five small box gardens (3x3 feet)

---

41. http://www.ewg.org/news/news-releases/2011/11/30/market-shift-hundreds-cosmetics-companies-fulfill-safe-products-pledge

where we plant a combination of a few veggies, herbs and flowers. The results are neat and healthful. We can pick greens for dinner, tomatoes for our salads, sweet basil as a garnish for the salads, and green beans in season. We use no pesticides so they're organic and they're freshly picked when we eat them. Not only are they good for our health and palate, but it's a pleasure to bask in the beauty of our backyard when we sit out on the patio in the evenings.

- If you can't grow it, buy organic produce at the grocery store, particularly with any of the "dirty dozen" veggies and fruits. If you can't buy organic produce, get commercially grown produce. It's better to get the nutritional benefit of these foods than to avoid them because of their pesticide exposure, but be sure to wash all produce well. Peel any fruits and veggies if they're from the "dirty dozen."

- Minimize purchase of highly processed foods. We get a few lightly processed foods such as packaged rice, steel-cut oats, and canned organic veggies and beans, but we avoid most heavily processed foods. I shop twice a week or more because we get so much fresh produce, but I spend very little time in the center aisles where most of the processed foods reside. It helps to shop from a grocery list. We write a list of what we need before I go to the store, and I follow this list almost exclusively.

- Avoid unnecessary x-ray exposure, especially from CT scans. Never ask your doctor for x-rays if he or she doesn't suggest them.

As we have seen, there are many complicated environmental issues. Regardless of the challenges involved, always look for positive solutions!

CHAPTER THIRTEEN

Caring Relationships

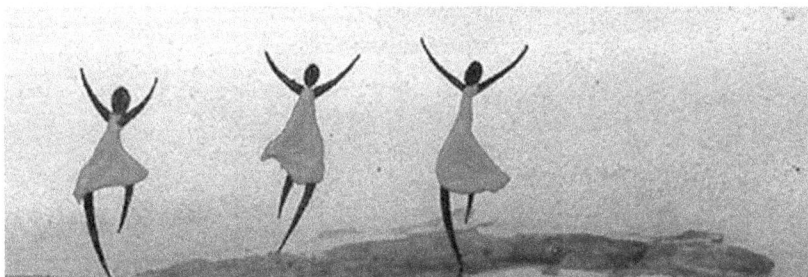

Caring for oneself may be considered selfish. Caring for others is sometimes considered sentimental foolishness in a world dominated by tough business interests. Yet, caring relationships are powerful determinants of health. Adam learns why they are so important in this chapter.

The Power of Caring Relationships

Healthy relationships are a vital part of a healthy lifestyle. We are biologically designed as social beings. Human babies are totally helpless when born. They die quickly without caring support, and they need nurturing for years before they can become independent. Love is an essential part of this support.

Studies in orphanages decades ago showed that infants did not thrive if they were not picked up with loving attention, even though they were bottle-fed and cleaned on schedule. Many died or developed serious physical, mental, and/or emotional problems as they grew. Loving care by a substitute mother changed these outcomes completely. Love made the difference.

Even as independent adults, humans need one another. "No man is an island, entire of itself; every man is a piece of the continent, a part of the main." These words, penned by John Donne four centuries ago, resonate more than ever today. Joan Baez's popular song of the 1960s echoes the same refrain.

Several decades ago, Dr. Dean Ornish showed that caring support was essential to help patients reverse severe heart disease. Healthy food, carefully supervised exercise, and meditation were all important parts of his program. Yet, in analyzing his data, he found that being members of caring support groups made the biggest difference of all. Love is our most powerful healing force.

Compassion, meaning "suffer with" or "empathize with," is similar to love in that it comes from the heart, but it avoids shades of meaning associated with the word love that are not relevant here. We'll look at why compassion for self and others is healthy, and what pitfalls it skirts. Then we'll look at how to nurture loving compassion as a way to strengthen healthy relationships.

Self-Compassion

In 2011, I was privileged to attend a workshop on Mindful Self-Compassion, led by Kristin Neff, PhD, Associate Professor in Human Development at the University of Texas. She wrote the book, *Self-Compassion*, based on ground-breaking research she has done on this subject over the past decade, The workshop was excellent, and her book is a valuable resource.

Early in her career, she focused on self-esteem, thinking it was one of the best ways to help people achieve their potential. Self-esteem is an important concept, but psychologists have begun to see flaws in it. It has been emphasized as a personal strength for decades in psychology but the benefits desired are not always obtained. It's worth exploring some of the reasons for this.

Most people think of themselves as above average. Psychologists call this the "Lake Wobegon" effect (for Garrison Keillor's famous fictional town where "all the women are strong, all the men are good-looking, and all the children are above average.") Real life surveys show that 85 percent of children think they are above average, and 90 percent of all drivers think they are more skilled than other drivers.[42]

The problem is that it's impossible for everybody to be above average. People see themselves through rose-colored glasses, but may use gray glasses to see imperfections in others. Looking at the weaknesses of others can boost self-esteem by comparison, but it's not a healthy kind of perception. The distortions involved are harmful to all concerned.

Focusing on oneself can lead to self-centered narcissism. Self-esteem can depend on achieving success at any cost to bolster one's ego. Failure to reach desired goals can result in anger directed at oneself or others. Projecting negatives on others can lead to prejudice and bullying tendencies.

The classic story of Cinderella illustrates the differences between self-centered self-esteem, and compassionate self-care. The stepmother and stepsisters were full of self-esteem based on degrading others. They cast Cinderella into a lowly, ash-carrying, role. Even though Cinderella's life looked hopelessly mired in failure, she never lost hope. Compassionate self-care eventually brought her ultimate success.

Differences between self-esteem and self-compassion are subtle, but crucial. If self-esteem is gained by down-grading others, the personal psychological cost can be high. Depression and anxiety lurk in the wings, ready to beat the self up for any self-perceived failure. Self-compassion, on the other hand, nurtures a healthy kind of self-esteem by learning to view the self and others through a lens of loving-kindness.

People with self-compassion know that we all make mistakes. To be

42. Kristin Neff. *Self-Compassion* (New York, NY: HarperCollins, 2011), p. 20.

human is to be fallible. We don't expect babies to walk perfectly the first time they stand up. It is in falling and getting back up repeatedly that they learn to become good walkers. Experiences of failure teach us a lot. Instead of beating ourselves up over a failure, we can view it as a valuable lesson.

Willingness to risk failure, if not wildly reckless, can be a strength. Fear of failure tends to inhibit initiative, and if that fear is pervasive, it can hobble development. On the other hand, the willingness to try something new despite the risk of failure can be growth-enhancing in the long run. Thomas Edison claimed to have 99 failures for every success.

It's important to keep this basic understanding alive as we grow. Unhappily, many people become increasingly critical of themselves and others. They can be harsher on themselves or their children than anyone else would be. If such criticism is constant, it can become toxic, and make people feel inadequate no matter how successful they seem.

Much research shows that people learn and perform better with encouragement. Mindful self-compassion offers this kind of influence. It helps people encourage themselves in positive ways.[43] It also helps them show compassionate understanding to others.

Many people think of compassion as being "wimpy," but it's not. Compassion is much different than self-pity. Self-pity cries and wallows in the muck, never learning from the experience. Compassion says: "You fell, but that's OK. You're learning valuable lessons. Just pick yourself up and keep on going."

Self-compassion can also be confused with self-indulgence, but they're not the same. The self-indulgent person says to herself after falling: "This is too difficult and painful." Seeking comfort, she does not learn from her experience. The self-compassionate person rubs her bruises after a fall, but gets up and keeps going. Compassion doesn't criticize, evade, or make

43. Ibid., p. 16.

excuses. Rather than being a weakness, it's a strength.

Self-esteem nurtured through self-compassion is a healthy kind of esteem. Because it comes from the inside, there is no need to downgrade anyone else. It is truly the strongest kind of self-esteem that anyone can possess.

Compassion for Others

As I've already noted, it's human to make mistakes. Recognizing that we're all in the same boat, people who learn to forgive themselves for their mistakes also learn to be forgiving with others.

Who comes to mind when you hear that someone is compassionate? You may think of someone who cares for others in their work, such as a nurse, or perhaps someone like Mother Teresa, who devoted her life to caring for the poor. Such associations are natural, but compassion is not restricted to full-time care-givers. We all have the seeds of compassion within us, even though we may not always nourish them.

The story of the Good Samaritan highlights this. A man was on the road to Jericho when robbers attacked him, stripped and beat him up, and left him half dead. A priest who came by saw him lying there, but passed by on the other side of the road. A Levite came by and did the same thing. Then a Samaritan came down the road, and when he saw the beaten man, his heart was filled with compassion. He treated the man's wounds, lifted him onto his own donkey, and carried him to the nearest inn. There, he arranged for the man's care.[44]

In this story, it's noteworthy that it was an ordinary man who showed compassion, not the religiously elite. Jesus made this contrast clear. The Samaritan belonged to a disdained faith and culture. In telling this story,

---

44. Luke 10: 30-35, *Good News Bible*, second edition, (The United Bible Societies, 1994).

Jesus made two subtle, but profound points. Everyone is of value, and nobody should be looked down upon—not those who have suffered ill-fortune, and not those who are culturally different. Compassion goes deeper than cultural convention.

Is there a risk of becoming overwhelmed with the needs of others to the point of being "burned-out?" Yes, there's danger of burn-out if a person doesn't take time to care for themselves. Compassion for others must be balanced by wise self-care. Reserving as little as ten minutes a day for quiet time to meditate and be open to God's loving wisdom makes all the difference in the world. This wisdom helps to keep one in good balance.

How we handle our relationships to others has a bearing on our health. The Grant Study was a longitudinal study of Harvard men from the classes of 1942, 1943, and 1944. It is still ongoing, though many of the men have now died. Dr. George Vaillant, co-director of the study, found that relationships to others predicted late-life adjustment better than most other factors. When asked what the study taught him, he said: "The only thing that really matters in life are your relationships to other people."

There is a biological reason why warm connections with others are good for health.[45] Oxytocin, sometimes called the love hormone, is released when people are engaged in caring behavior. It promotes bonding between people. Its levels rise with activities ranging from simple hugging, to enjoying meals together, to cherishing thoughts about a loved one.

Oxytocin secretion rises in women and their babies during labor, peaking with natural delivery. Breast-feeding also stimulates release of oxytocin. It is no wonder that the mother-child bond is strong, but it's not the only bond. Some level of bonding is involved in all caring relationships.[46]

---

45. http://www.heartmath.com/articles/altruism-stress-remedy.html

46. http://psychcentral.com/lib/about-oxytocin/0001386

The heart has oxytocin receptors, and it goes into a harmonious rhythm when a person simply thinks about any experience of caring or being cared for.[47] The evidence is abundant that a spirit of caring promotes health and happiness.

Doing Fun Things Together

A popular saying goes, "The family that plays together stays together." One commentator writes that having fun together is at the top of his list for promoting family health. Others note that laughing together strengthens family bonds. Going to favorite locations for family vacation times can build a strong sense of family unity. Simply being engaged in doing fun things together nourishes the family.

When I was a teenager and our family was living in New Jersey, dad and mom established the tradition of having a family game night every Friday night. After dinner, we gathered in the family room to play various kinds of games, ranging from board games like Parcheesi or Monopoly, to family card games like Rook. Halfway through the evening, Dad would wash and quarter some apples for us to munch on, and then we'd finish whatever game we were playing.

I don't remember details of those evenings such as who won or lost, but I do recall them as fun evenings that we all enjoyed. We had no car or TV. We were poor in material wealth (missionary families didn't earn much money,) but we were rich in family togetherness, and that meant a lot.

One relationship caution to keep in mind about games is that an over-emphasis on winning is not wise. The value of having fun together is in strengthening connections. If a game is one of winning at all costs, it can destroy the value of playing together. If a winning strategy involves cheating,

---

47. http://bellybelly.com.au/birth/ecstatic-birth-natures-hormonal-blueprint-for-labor

or if "one-upmanship" becomes the name of the game, unhealthy anger or depression may be the result instead of a feeling of camaraderie.

Going to Source

We've reviewed the value of healthy relationships with oneself and others, but there's one more relationship to look at. That is the relationship we have with our creator. In discussing this, I'm assuming that we have a creative source and that it's possible to relate to this creative power in some way. Some people don't agree with these assumptions, and that's OK. If you don't agree, this section still has value for you, as you will see.

It's worth noting that not believing in a universal creative power takes faith, just as it does to believe in such a power. There is no proof of either the presence or the absence of God in the creation of the universe. The wonders of the universe makes many scientists think it's less likely that it came about by chance than that there's a creative power at work. Believing in chance is as much a matter of faith as believing in God.

If one accepts the possibility of a universal creative power, how does one relate to that power? The classic way of doing this is through prayer and meditation. Without delving into the mystery of how prayer or meditation help us connect with our creative source, let's look at the evidence that meditation is helpful to those who use it.

The first scientific evidence that a process similar to meditation is helpful to users was established by Dr. Herbert Benson at Harvard University in the early 1970s. Benson studied the relaxation response, as he labeled it, to see if it brought about any benefits. In carefully designed studies with volunteers, he documented solid evidence that it was effective in reducing stress, lowering blood pressure, and reducing other risks to health.

His ground-breaking book, *The Relaxation Response,* published in 1975, helped establish the value of mind-body medicine, and it has become a classic. Although he called his technique "the relaxation response" to avoid religious connotations, the process involved is similar to most meditative practices.

Subjects are asked to close their eyes and focus on slowing their breathing as they mentally repeat a simple word or phrase, such as "Peace." They do this for ten to fifteen minutes once or twice a day. The relief from stress provided by this simple process is very effective.

Over the years, *The Relaxation Response* has sold over four million copies. It gained scientific acceptance because Benson documented his research very thoroughly, and because his approach was secular. His book and method is still highly recommended by many physicians and psychologists for its therapeutic value.[48]

Since then, other researchers have documented many benefits of meditation. Perhaps the most intriguing research is by Dr. Richard Davidson at the University of Wisconsin. His laboratory established the fact that meditation produces changes in brain structure as well as benefits to a person's health. His new book, titled *The Emotional Life of Your Brain*, is a good summary of his research on emotions and the brain.[49]

Davidson and other researchers have learned that the brain is structurally more changeable than we ever knew before. We can change our brains physically by the way we think, live, and meditate. The long-term benefits of meditation are good for us at many levels, physically, mentally, and emotionally.

Janet Conner penned the book, *Writing Down Your Soul*, a best-seller in its genre. My wife and I took a week-long workshop with Janet on how to bring writing into meditative practice. Held in Oaxaca, Mexico, the setting was wonderful for learning about Zapotec history and culture, but the

48. http://www.relaxationresponse.org/

49. http://richardjdavidson.com/research/

deepest impact for me came from Janet's classes where I learned this new way of enhancing my meditation time.

Janet wrote her book out of her own soul-searing experience. She describes the desperation she felt as her life fell apart when her husband deserted her. Yet it was in that dark night of the soul that she discovered the power of pouring out her emotions in writing. Her practice of writing down her soul's deepest feelings grew out of that experience.[50]

Although my story is not dramatic, I've found that "writing down my soul" enriches my life in a new way. The insights and guidance I receive sometimes amaze me. Even if I don't gain any specific insight, I feel connected to a source of wisdom that is deeper than any conscious wisdom I possess.

Many studies document the value of journaling, whether done in connection with meditation or not. Benefits include stress reduction, healing, self discovery, problem solving, growth, and enhanced creativity, among others. This is very similar to the benefits of meditation. Writing is not essential for effective meditation, but it helps.

Jesus advised going into one's closet to pray rather than praying on the street corner. In this inner sanctum, free of external distractions, one is most open to hearing the still small voice of God. Meditation and writing down one's soul are simply other ways of opening up to this inner voice.

A healthy relationship with universal source is important on its own merits, but it's also basic to having a healthy relationship with one's neighbor and oneself. All three kinds of relationship are essential for healthy, vibrant, living.

---

50. http://www.janetconner.com

CHAPTER FOURTEEN

Health and Well-Being

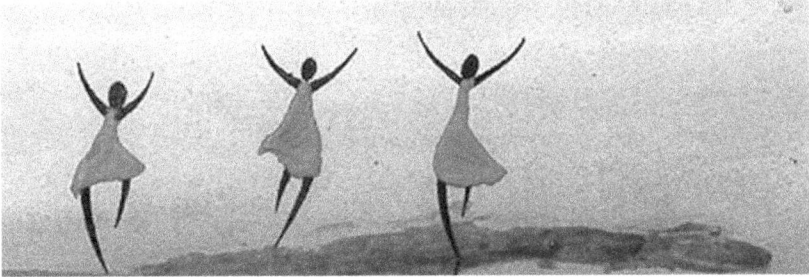

Health and well-being are states of being that most people desire. Although they sound similar, there are differences between them. Health has been well-defined, but surprisingly, there is considerable controversy about a definition for well-being. In this chapter, Adam gains some understanding about this, and begins to see how health and well-being are mutually reinforcing.

Health and Well-Being

Health and well-being are connected in some ways, but the relationship is complex. One can have a sense of well-being in spite of health problems. Conversely, one can be in good general health, but lack an overall sense of well-being. Health is an important facet of well-being, but well-being is broader than health. It involves a sense of purpose that adds depth and meaning to life. Because of this, it's worth taking time to look a little more deeply into well-being.

Viktor Frankl's book, *Man's Search for Meaning*, is about life and survival in a Nazi concentration camp in World War II. Even in that horrific setting, a few people found meaning through simple acts of kindness. Frankl saw that those able to find some meaning in their lives, even in the concentration camp, were most likely to survive. The importance of man's search for meaning was at the heart of his method of psychotherapy.[51]

Positive Psychology

Research studies carried out in the past 20 years confirm that a sense of purpose is essential to positive living. Positive psychology has come to the fore in the past 20 years. Almost totally neglected before that, thousands of studies now confirm its value. Martin Seligman, called the father of positive psychology, writes that purpose is vital to well-being. In his book, *Flourish*, he shows that purpose, engagement, relationships, meaning, and accomplishment are all important to a positive sense of well-being.[52]

Barbara Fredrickson, in her book, *Positivity*, says that having a positive outlook does more to build success than anything else. Uplifting qualities such as gratitude, serenity, hope, and love, among others, are positive. Over the past 20 years, Dr. Fredrickson has probed the impact of both positive and negative emotions. Her research, involving thousands of people in many different studies, shows how much positivity contributes to successful living.[53] A widely recognized leader in this field, her findings have been reinforced by the work of many other scientists.

In contrast to positivity, pervasive negativity is unfavorable in its impact on life and health. It can dominate one's self-talk and judgments, causing health-damaging emotions such as depression, contempt, and anger. These affect the entire body, raising blood pressure, tensing muscles throughout

51. Viktor E. Frankl, MD. *Man's Search for Meaning*, Updated Edition (New York, NY: Pocket Books, 1997).

52. Martin Seligman, E.P. PhD. *Flourish*, Reprint Edition (New York, NY: Free Press, 2011).

53. Barbara L. Fredrickson, PhD. *Positivity*, (New York, NY: Three Rivers Press, 2009).

the body, and causing corrosive damage to many physiological functions.

Psychologists have long known that negative emotions affect the mind and body more strongly than positive emotions. Because negativity bias is dominant, most past research in this field has studied negative emotional life to see if it can be effectively treated or neutralized. Research in the past two decades on the value of positivity reveals that nurturing a positive mental and emotional outlook is more effective than simply trying to treat entrenched negative emotions.

The "Tipping Point"

An interesting research finding is that a ratio of three positive thoughts to one negative thought is important. Fredrickson calls this ratio the "tipping point." Those who consistently have a positivity ratio above 3:1 are more likely to be resilient and successful. The 3:1 ratio forecasts success in many areas, including marriage, business, sports, and much else. The research shows that this ratio predicts success rather than being the result of success.

Why is the 3:1 ratio so effective? Fredrickson's research suggests that it takes this much positivity to pull free from negativity's downward push. People who stay above the tipping point have broader perspectives and are more open to new ideas and experiences. Because of these qualities, they are more likely to be productive in many ways. Brain imaging shows that their brain structures and activity are enhanced at vital centers of connectivity. This correlates with their ability to make many productive associations in life.

Only one of every five people tested have 3:1 positivity ratios or better. Four out of five people live with lower ratios. Those with ratios around 2:1 may do fairly well, but still fail to reach their full potential. Those with ratios of 1:1 or lower are most likely to suffer from serious depression.

Negatives have some value. Falls in life are inevitable. Sadness, grief, and anger can be cathartic. Positive growth emerging from negative experiences is possible. Forged steel is stronger than iron is as a base metal. Resilience shaped by difficult experiences can strengthen a person. Still, it's not good to be swamped by negativity. Having a predominantly positive outlook on life is most valuable.

The good news is that people can raise their positivity ratios. A person's perspective can shift from seeing the glass of life half empty, to seeing it half full; from seeing darkness, to seeing rays of hope. People deficient in positivity can learn to become more positive. This has to be more than superficial change. Fake positivity does not work. You must develop genuine inner positivity to experience real change in life. So, how do you go about building authentic positivity? The first step is to learn your own positivity ratio.

The Positivity Self Test

Fredrickson has developed a "Positivity Self Test" so anyone can check his or her own positivity ratio. It is free on her website for anyone to take. The test is easy to complete, consisting of a series of 20 questions about the feelings one has experienced that day. There are five possible responses for each question. Test-takers choose a response for each question that reflects their feelings most accurately.

The questions must be answered as honestly as possible. Fake positivity has no value, so there's no reason to give false answers. It only takes a few minutes to complete the test. When finished, click the "Submit" button, and wait for the answer. Within a minute, a report with your calculated positivity ratio pops up on the screen. That's how quickly you can find out where you stand on the positivity scale.

A single test result is worth getting, but Fredrickson emphasizes that test results are best if repeated daily for two weeks. That's because feelings normally fluctuate from day to day, so a two-week average test score provides a better baseline than a test score from a single day. I can confirm this from my own test results. Anyone wishing to take the test can do so at the following website: http://www.positivityratio.com/single.php

In addition to creating the Positivity Self Test, Fredrickson has also developed a Positivity Toolkit for anyone wanting to strengthen his or her positivity traits. She has tested this toolkit extensively, providing solid evidence that it works for those who put it to good use.[54]

The Positivity Toolkit has a dozen "tools" to help counter negativity and strengthen positivity. I'll discuss a few of these tools to give you an idea of what they are like. They include appreciating nature, developing a gratitude ritual, cultivating kindness, and learning to practice mindful meditation. Appreciating nature can be as simple as walking to a neighborhood park or spending time in your own yard.

My two-year-old grandson taught me something about nature appreciation when I took him for a walk in our yard a few years ago. Every step or two, he bent down to examine a blade of grass, a new little weed, an acorn cap or a little stone. He showed me each new find with great excitement. We didn't walk far that hour, but we truly appreciated nature!

Gratitude is a strong reinforcer of positivity. In addition to thanking others for small or great kindnesses, it's worth developing the habit of writing down a brief list of three or four things you are grateful for each day. I write down thanks in my meditation journal each day for three blessings that I experience. This can be done anytime, and it doesn't have to be in a journal. The value comes from taking a moment to think of people, events, or experiences one is grateful for. Writing down one's gratitude strongly reinforces its benefits in the mind.

Cultivating kindness is not a difficult task. It's mainly a matter of being

---

54. Ibid., pp 199-223.

aware of small things one can do to help others. This can be as simple as helping to clean up after a meal or giving someone a genuine smile. The value lies in the mental attitude as much as in the act of kindness. As a side-note, notice how much a genuine smile beautifies anyone's face. It's a benefit for both giver and receiver!

Meditation helps build positivity, although that's not its primary purpose. I discussed meditation in chapter eleven, so I won't repeat myself. Still, it's worth emphasizing that spending as little as ten minutes a day to quietly meditate helps immensely in navigating through the rest of the day. The benefits may seem minor at first, but as time goes by, they grow in value. Eventually, the benefits of meditation can be powerful indeed.

For a full discussion of the Positivity Toolkit, I highly recommend reading Fredrickson's book, *Positivity*. Learning about various facets of positivity reviewed by Fredrickson is worthwhile. The chapters on the Self Test and the Positivity Toolkit alone are worth the price of the book. Following Fredrickson's guidance is an excellent way to help build a strong foundation for personal growth and development.

Positivity and Well-Being

Research done by Martin Seligman, Barbara Fredrickson and others, shows that positivity is strongly correlated with well-being. Seligman's criteria for well-being include five components, the first of which is positive emotion. This is deeper and more enduring than happiness, which can come and go. Most people desire happiness, but it is an elusive concept that can be hard to pin down.

Thomas Jefferson said the pursuit of happiness was one of the basic rights of man, but he did not mean the pursuit of pleasure that drives many people. To Jefferson, happiness included a quality of self-restraint that helped one reach fulfillment. That differs from an idea of happiness based on pleasure that may be short-lived. To avoid confusion over the meaning of happiness, Seligman prefers the phrase, *positive emotion.* Even with this broader label, Seligman says it is only one of five elements that make up well-being.

The other elements of well-being include engagement, relationships, meaning, and accomplishment. Each element is significant by itself, but they are even stronger when combined. *Engagement* means being deeply involved in something, not simply skimming its surface. *Meaning* serves a purpose deeper than frittering away time. *Accomplishment* involves the sense of mastering any skill or goal.

Positive relationships are important for many reasons. Biologically, we are social beings. Many biologists today say there is much evidence to suggest that the group, rather than the individual, is the primary unit of natural selection. Emotionally, we are relationship oriented, and research shows this to be so important that Seligman classifies it as one of the basic elements of well-being.

All of this is significant with regard to health. Most people want to enjoy positive health, physically, mentally, and emotionally. People who are fully engaged in finding the best ways to work toward their goals are more likely to succeed than those who make only a few superficial efforts before giving up. People who support each other toward their goals do better than people who feel isolated. The accomplishment that comes from working together helps build motivation. Good health and well-being are mutually reinforcing.

Money and Well-Being

Is there a relationship between money and well-being? If so, what is the relationship, and how strong is it? I touched on this issue in an earlier chapter, but it's worth re-visiting. Seligman explores this question in his book, *Flourishing*. Many other psychologists, sociologists, and economists have also explored this question. Clearly, it is an important question that interests many people.[55]

The consensus from this research seems to be that there is a relationship between money and well-being, but it is a limited relationship. If one lacks the resources to supply basic needs (such as adequate food, shelter, and clothing,) money to supply those needs is helpful for well-being. After basic needs are met, the money/well-being relationship is complex. Money remains useful, but there is less correlation between income and well-being.

The drive to accumulate ever more wealth is not a guarantee of happiness or well-being. A quote attributed to Franklin D. Roosevelt speaks to this point. "Happiness lies not in the mere possession of money; it lies in the joy of achievement, in the thrill of creative effort."

Interestingly enough, cross-cultural surveys show that some countries with lower than average incomes have higher happiness indices some high income countries. Again, this suggests that the relationship between income and well-being is limited. Columnist Gregg Easterbrook writes many perceptive essays. A paragraph in one titled, *The Real Truth About Money*, is worth quoting here.

"There is a final reason money can't buy happiness: the things that really matter in life are not sold in stores. Love, friendship, family, respect, a place in the community, the belief that your life has purpose—those are the essentials of human fulfillment, and they cannot be purchased with cash. Everyone needs a certain amount of money, but chasing money rather than meaning is a formula for discontent. Too many Americans have made materialism and the cycle of 'work and spend' their principal goals. Then

55. http://knowledge.wharton.upenn.edu/article/gross-domestic-happiness-what-is-the-relationship-between-money-and-well-being/

they wonder why they don't feel happy."[56]

National Well-Being

In his book, *Flourishing*, Dr. Seligman recommends measuring national progress in terms of well-being rather than economic growth. He points out that much of our Gross Domestic Product (GDP) includes things that are not positive for well-being. Money spent on jails, car wrecks, and illicit drugs do not contribute to well-being, but all such expenditures are bundled into our GDP as growth indicators.

The concept of making national well-being a goal, and measuring it annually to check our progress sounds idealistic, but it is not an impossibility. Measurable indicators of well-being are possible. British Prime Minister David Cameron announced plans in November, 2010 to measure well-being in the UK. He officially asked the Office of National Statistics (ONS) to initiate public discussion about this project, and then develop plans to begin measuring it.[57]

In response, the ONS began to develop a range of **well-being indicators** to measure "happiness, life satisfaction, and purpose in life" that will be included in national household surveys.[58] Commenting on David Cameron's initiative, the New Economics Foundation (NEF) in Britain agrees that people's well-being is what should be measured and used to guide national policy.

It states that the economy is a means to an end, and not to be valued as an end in itself. It is significant insofar as it contributes to happy and healthy

---

56. http://www.time.com/time/magazine/article/0,9171,1015883,00.html#ixzz1fVLKmkwa

57. http://www.ons.gov.uk/ons/guide-method/user-guidance/well-being/index.html

58. Ibid.

fulfilled lives. NEF goes on to say that this focus on well-being should be combined with an emphasis on sustainability of the earth's resources. Sustainable well-being is vital for both society and the planet.[59]

It is beyond the scope of this book to analyze national well being, but a few comments are worth making. The first point is that well-being is receiving national and international attention as an achievable goal worth pursuing. It is not being waved off as a "pie-in-the-sky" idea.

The second point is that while well-being and optimal health are not identical concepts, they are closely intertwined at both the individual and the national levels. Working toward either one helps boost the other one. To underline this point, if healthy lifestyles became standard in the USA, the new standard would transform individual lives across the nation and enhance national well-being at the same time.

The degree to which this could renew our nation is hard to estimate, but it would be substantial. The potential for improvement in the health care field alone is astonishing. It is estimated that over half of the common chronic diseases in the USA are preventable. If half of the cases of type 2 diabetes, hypertension, heart disease, obesity, and cancer were prevented over the next few years, improvements in well-being at all levels would be great. As a side benefit, there would be great savings in national health care costs.

One final comment on the topic of national well-being: It's fine for any government to establish a policy of encouraging optimal health and well-being, but it's important to avoid forcing these goals on people. Any sense of requiring people to strive for such goals is self-defeating. A policy of making these goals attractive so that people want to reach them is better by far. The rewards of healthy living are attractive on their own. If people understood how significant these rewards are, they would go to the ends of the earth to find them. Fortunately, they don't have to go that far. They

---

59. http://www.neweconomics.org/issues/entry/well-being

only have to look within to find the resources they need.

The Joys of Well-Being

This book is about discovering the power and joy to be found in healthy living. Some people equate healthy living with a boring, spartan way of life. The truth is that healthy living is a joy. A certain degree of self-discipline is involved to be sure, but it is far from boring. In concluding this chapter, let's look at some of the joys of healthy living.

First, there is the enriching joy of healthy relationships. Most people can remember the joy that small children express when they are happy. It kindles joy in those around them when they squeal in delight at a new discovery, or in finding something or someone they love. I'm always impressed by how much fun toddlers have with a new achievement, such as climbing up on a chair, or in playing a familiar game like peek-a-boo or hide-and-seek. Their peals of laughter at being found are pure celebration of the joy of life.

Adults may be more restrained in expressing their joy, but ongoing friendships and reconnection with old friends are sources of joy that most people experience. Family ties are nourishing across miles of separation and generations of life. One of the joys of grandparenthood is rediscovering the joys of childhood as they play with their grandchildren. Healthy relationships provide lifelong fountains of joy.

Exercise is a wonderful way of generating joyful energy. Small children exhibit this when they run and play with inexhaustible energy, but it's true for all ages. Teenagers playing sports like soccer, basketball, and tennis; young adults dancing the night away; and older folks taking enjoyable walks together: All are reaping benefits of exercise. Healthy exercise is simply a wonderful way to express the joy of life.

Enjoyment of the environment adds richness to the joy of healthy living. Canoeing across a pristine sparkling lake, vibrantly alive with darting fish, paddling ducks, and colorful shorebirds, is a soul-stirring experience. Climbing mountain trails to reach remote waterfalls is exhilarating. Hiking high coastal trails with wonderful views of soaring gulls and the pounding surf below are awe-inspiring. Visiting a park or simply sitting under a tree are gentle ways of enjoying creation. Nature's cleansing and filtering processes work wonders everywhere.

Gardening is a joy for me, as it is for millions. Spading, sifting soil through my fingers, and planting seeds in the good earth feels good. Watching the seedlings sprout and grow into the unique plants they're meant to be is awesome: Colorful beet greens with deep red beets; graceful lacy pea vines with delicate white flowers and beautiful green pods; hearty zucchini plants with magnificent umbrella-like leaves and gorgeous yellow blossoms; and the startling white stems and bright green leaves of bok choy. Soil, sun and rain nourish this DNA-guided diversity. It is a miracle of nature.

Harvesting abundant fruits and veggies is another joy. Eating delicately steamed greens, delicious sweet peas, and sweet corn-on-the-cob is a wonderful sensory experience. Aside from their great nutritional value, the taste of fresh, ripe, organic vegetables and fruit simply can't be matched. Even in the city, our small garden beds are spaces of joy.

Research confirms that a healthy lifestyle adds years to life. It also adds life to those years. It's not the years as much as the joy in them that is the blessing. The joy of healthy living is not a "pie-in-the-sky" theory. It is the real deal. Well-being is the reward of the life well lived, physically, mentally, spiritually and emotionally.

CHAPTER FIFTEEN

The Power of Lifestyle

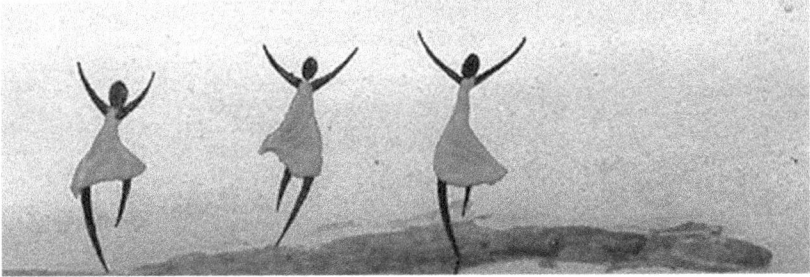

The power of lifestyle is greater than most people realize, both for good and for bad. If someone has lifestyle factors that aren't healthy, such as eating lots of junk foods, watching too much television (several hours daily), smoking, or not engaging in regular physical activity, the negative impact of these lifestyle factors on health is huge. Conversely, if a person's lifestyle factors are healthy, the positive impact of these factors is great. For better or worse, your lifestyle is very powerful in shaping the quality of your health!

Lifestyle and Health

Your lifestyle is more powerful in determining the overall quality of your health than almost anything else. It's more powerful than your genes, your doctors, your pills, or your income, though all of these certainly influence your health. Three stories vividly illustrate the power of lifestyle.

The Health-Sabotaging Lifestyle

Frank was a 39-year old man who came into the hospital because of experiencing crushing chest pain. He had suffered a previous heart attack before, but this one was worse. Coronary arteriography revealed that he had severe coronary artery disease, so severe that our cardiology consultants said that he was not a candidate for heart surgery.

Frank was frightened, knowing that his life hung in the balance. The ways of life he had followed for many years had to change if he wanted to survive. He had smoked two or three packs of cigarettes daily for over 20 years. He did not engage in any regular exercise. He described himself as a "meat and potatoes" man, rarely eating any kind of veggies or fruit. Finally, his relationships with most people were poor because of his abrasive personality.

After being in the Critical Care Unit for several days, Frank improved enough to be moved to a semi-private room. He received gentle cardiac rehab and dietary counseling. I spent considerable time with him making sure he understood how crucial it was for him to follow his program. He said he would take his medications and follow his rehab program. Before leaving the hospital, he also promised me that he would not resume smoking.

When Frank kept his first appointment to see me a week later, he was smoking again. He failed all his appointments after that. When I called to find out why he was not coming to see me or going to cardiac rehab, his wife told me, "Doc, you might as well be talking to the wall when you talk with Frank. He's not going to change." She would have been supportive if he had been willing, but he wasn't, and after years of living with him, she simply gave me her realistic assessment.

Less than six months later, Frank came into the hospital Emergency Department with his third major heart attack. He did not survive this one, never making it out of the Emergency Department. His death at age 39 was not the youngest ever recorded for severe coronary artery disease, but he died far younger than he should have. (Frank is a fictitious name, but his story is real.)

The Health-Empowering Lifestyle

Ralph was a missionary in Angola, Africa who suffered many attacks of malaria there, even though he took quinine, the main medication for malaria at that time. At age 32 he developed a complication of malaria called blackwater fever, so called because the urine turns black from the massive destruction of red blood cells caused by the malaria parasites. Blackwater fever is still dreaded because its fatality rates remain high.

A veteran missionary sat at Ralph's bedside for 24 hours, forcing him to drink a glass of water every fifteen minutes. She told him that keeping his kidneys functioning by forcing fluids was his main hope of surviving. Thanks to her dedicated perseverance, he survived, and eventually he regained his normal strength and resilience.

Aside from the risk of malaria due to his work in Africa, his way of life was healthy. He grew up on a farm in Iowa and his parents always had a great garden. Ralph grew up eating lots of vegetables and fruit, and he worked hard on the farm. Later, he always planted a garden wherever he lived. In addition to the good produce it provided, it gave him plenty of exercise as well as a chance to enjoy his little corner of God's world.

Ralph was the first of his family to go to college, and then to seminary. He related well to those around him, and he was someone who could be relied upon completely. His word was his bond. When he was 90 years old, he was invited to return to Africa to speak and participate in the Centennial celebration of Methodism in Africa. While there, he was also awarded an honorary doctorate by Africa University.

At age 98, Ralph still spent several hours a day working in his garden, growing abundant produce for the table. He ate mainly vegetarian meals with occasional fish or chicken, and his appetite was excellent. His weight was ideal for his age, his blood pressure was excellent, and his blood tests were all normal. He did not require any medication. Unfortunately, he had mild Alzheimer's disease the last three years of his life. He died in a home setting at age 101. I knew Ralph well because he was my father.

A Lifestyle Turn-Around

Robert was 61 years old when his frequent "indigestion" flared up in January 2008. His internist gave him a careful examination, and then advised an exercise nuclear heart scan. Robert could only stay on the treadmill for six minutes before becoming totally exhausted and experiencing the same kind of "indigestion" pain he had been having frequently. This time it was worse.

Robert wasn't surprised when his doctor said his test showed evidence of heart trouble and referred him to a cardiologist, but it was a wake-up call. Even though he enjoyed kayaking and thought himself to be in average health, he weighed 250 pounds and was on pills for high blood pressure, high cholesterol, and diabetes.

While waiting for his cardiology appointment, Robert researched the internet to find out how he might help himself. There he learned that lifestyle changes recommended by physicians such as Dr. John McDougall and Dr. Caldwell Esselstyn could help him. What he learned about Dr. Esselstyn's holistic program at the Cleveland Clinic impressed him. He decided he wanted to follow it if his internist and cardiologist said OK to the idea.

When the cardiologist saw Robert and reviewed all his reports, he explained that the stress test revealed significant heart wall abnormality due to poor blood supply. He advised x-rays of the coronary arteries and probable stent placement to improve the blood supply to his heart muscle. Robert said he understood, but asked if he could have a trial period with diet and medical management first. His doctors were not keen about this idea, but they finally agreed.

Robert followed Dr. Esselstyn's program very carefully. When he saw his cardiologist one year later, he was a revitalized edition of his former self. He had lost 60 pounds. His blood pressure, cholesterol level, and blood sugar had all returned to normal levels, and his internist had gradually taken him off all his medications as his health improved. When Robert repeated the cardiac stress test, he was able to go a full ten minutes on the treadmill with no symptoms.

His improvement puzzled the cardiologist. He said the abnormal heart weakness had cleared up, but implied that there must have been some error on the first test. Skeptically, he asked Robert if he had really given his best effort the first time. Robert told him he had. While the cardiologist was a skeptic, Robert's internist was impressed. He had monitored Robert's progress carefully, adjusting his medications when needed, and he knew that Robert's improvement was real.[60]

Robert's story is revealing on three levels. On a personal level, it shows how a deeply motivated person can dramatically turn his health around by making effective lifestyle changes. The turn-around in Robert's physical health was dramatic, but it took an equally major change in his mindset to allow this.

On a second level, the reaction of the cardiologist to the changes in Robert's health reveals how deeply enmeshed he was in the rescue model of health care. His mind was so closed to the obvious improvements in front of his own eyes that a faulty test was the only explanation he would consider.

On yet a third level, Robert's story shows the need to transform our model of health care to harmonize it with our evolving understanding of health. Many medical treatment outcomes are now surpassed by those associated with lifestyle medicine.

60. http://www.drmcdougall.com/misc/2009stars/robert2.htm
(Note: Robert tells his own story on the internet at this website.)

The Rescue Model of Health Care

The rescue model of health care is the main model of care in the Western world today. It focuses on rescuing people who are struggling with their health. It has major accomplishments to its credit. Yet, it also has a serious flaw.

Over the past century, as medical care became more sophisticated and medical practitioners more skilled at treating the many chronic diseases that began to overwhelm the Western world, it was natural that increasing emphasis was placed on diagnosis and treatment. Patients with heart failure, high blood pressure, stroke, and diabetes needed immediate care. Urgently needed treatment produced faster results and seemed more effective than prevention.

The result was the creation of magnificent treatment centers that are splendid showcases of medical care. Why is this a problem? Excellent care is not the problem, but pouring major resources, energy, and talent into this kind of treatment approach while investing only a small fraction of our resources in the prevention of these diseases was not wise.

Prevention was not totally neglected. We saw the birth of excellent centers of public health and preventive research such as the Johns Hopkins School of Hygiene and Public Health, among others. We also saw great progress in the fight to prevent many infectious diseases. Prevention was not overlooked. Yet, resources dedicated to prevention were a pittance compared to the resources devoted to treatment.

The emergence of chronic diseases such as coronary artery disease, stroke, type 2 diabetes, hypertension, cancer, and other major killers stimulated treatment more than prevention. Yet, we now know these diseases are largely preventable. We developed very expensive treatments such as coronary artery bypass surgery, but we could have prevented about 75 percent of these underlying diseases from occurring in the first place.

Our medical care system is a massive rescue system, with skilled specialists snatching millions of people from the danger of imminent death. They do marvelous work in saving people's lives and rebuilding damaged bodies. Yet, our magnificent medical centers are literally built on an unhealthy foundation. Most of the drama and suffering could be prevented. We know today that healthy lifestyles can prevent most of these chronic diseases.

Robert's case is not isolated. Thousands of patients have experienced similar benefits under the guidance of physicians like Dr. Dean Ornish, Dr. Caldwell Esselstyn, Dr. Joel Fuhrman, Dr. John McDougall, and other pioneers in the practice of lifestyle medicine. Their work in helping patients with severe life-threatening disease regain good health outshines all that the best in the rescue paradigm can offer.

Today, there is growing recognition of the importance of a healthy lifestyle. Groups like the American College of Lifestyle Medicine are spreading this message. Yet, we have a long way to go. Overall, our health care system is not geared up to provide solid directions for healthy living. An extremely expensive medical rescue system still dominates health care today. Major players in this system recognize that change is essential.

Mainstream Medicine Recognizes the Importance of Lifestyle Choices

More and more good research articles in leading medical journals discuss lifestyle as an important factor in determining health outcomes in their research. An article in the *Journal of the American Medical Association* (JAMA) in April, 2013, reported an international study of 153,996 adults carried out from 2003 through 2009 in seventeen countries. Of those enrolled in the study, 7,519 suffered a heart event or stroke event.

The study found that a low percentage of individuals with heart disease or stroke followed three key behaviors being analyzed, namely not smoking, being physically active, and following a healthy diet. Over three times that many did not follow any of these healthy practices.

This pattern of failing to practice healthy behavior was evident worldwide, especially in poorer countries. The authors noted that lifestyle changes to reduce the risk of recurrent events are essential, but that current efforts to modify such behavior are only modestly effective. They concluded that development of effective and low-cost prevention strategies are required.[61]

The Cost of Diabetes in the United States

A program titled "Unique Perspectives on the Cost Burden of Diabetes in the United States" was released on the Internet on July 31, 2013. A distinguished panel of physicians in leadership positions with the American Diabetes Association and in academic medicine reviewed the issue of how to best address the huge burden of diabetes in the USA today. One-fifth of health care dollars and one-third of Medicare dollars are now spent on diabetes in the USA.

The crux of the problem is that more people than ever have diabetes. After discussing all aspects of this problem, panelists agreed that prevention is key to improving this situation.

Dr. Sergio Fazio, Professor of Medicine at Vanderbilt University School of Medicine, said that lifestyle choices and obesity are the underlying problem in most cases. He added that society must recognize these issues as the basic problem in many of our current diseases. He concluded that improvement in dealing with obesity and poor lifestyle choices is needed to help prevent diabetes.[62] All the other panelists agreed with him.

---

61. http://jama.jamanetwork.com/article.aspx?articleid=1679401

62. http://www.medscape.org/viewarticle/808527_transcript

The State of US Health

A major analysis, titled "The State of US Health, 1990-2010: Burden of Diseases, Injuries, and Risk Factors," was published in the *Journal of the American Medical Association* on August 14, 2013. This massive study shows that the state of US Health improved a bit during this 20-year time span, but that in comparison to other wealthy countries, the USA did not keep pace.

The authors conclude that the best way for the US health care system to improve the nation's health would be to invest in public health programs and in multi-sectoral action to "address risks such as physical inactivity, diet, ambient particulate pollution, and alcohol and tobacco consumption."[63] Better lifestyle choices offer the best hope for helping to improve our national health.

These recent articles highlight the point that top medical authorities in medicine today understand the lifestyle choices people make are key factors determining their health. If we want to improve our health as a nation or as individuals, making healthy lifestyle choices is at the top of the list of what we can do for ourselves.

Are Lifestyle-related Health Problems Reversible?

Unfortunately, the disease-prone lifestyle is so deeply embedded in American and Western culture that it is viewed as being the norm. Being overweight and subject to high blood pressure, high cholesterol, cardio-vascular disease, diabetes, and arthritis after the age of 50 is so common that people often regard these health problems as simply part of the aging process. Few understand that they are largely preventable.

63. The State of US Health, 1990-2010. *Journal of the American Medical Association*. 2013; 310(6): 591-608.

The goal of good health is achievable for most people, and lifestyle is the master key to determine this. For millions of people who already have serious lifestyle-related health problems, a crucial question is, "Are these diseases reversible?" The answer is "Yes." They are reversible if patients adopt healthy living habits, and if the disease is caught before it is too far advanced.

Good studies show that type 2 diabetes, hypertension, high cholesterol, obesity, and even cardiovascular disease can be reversed with a healthy lifestyle. Cardiologist Dr. Dean Ornish proved that even advanced coronary artery disease can be reversed with his healthy living program. Dr. John McDougall has records of hundreds of patients with various chronic diseases whom he helped return to good health by teaching them the principles of a healthy lifestyle.

Nutritional, physical, and mental/emotional well-being are not stand-alone qualities. Good nutrition supports physical fitness. Both are integrally linked to mental/emotional wellness, which is linked to qualities of spirit like love, joy, and peace. All these relationships are reciprocal, working together to create an integrated, health-empowering lifestyle. They are more effective together than any of them are alone.

The earlier anyone adopts a healthy lifestyle, the better. If someone is traveling a health-damaging route, that person can change to a health-empowering course if motivated to do so before it's too late. This is good news for millions of people. Our nation would also benefit greatly from this kind of health revival.

Choose a Health-Empowering Lifestyle

Choosing a health-empowering lifestyle is clearly worthwhile. The tough question is how to make such change if it's needed. Changing long established habits of living is not easy. No single activity makes or breaks health by itself. It is the overall life pattern that is important. The more one's pattern is based on a healthy lifestyle, the better overall health is likely to be.

A healthy lifestyle is not complicated. It doesn't take genius to figure it out. Most people know that good food, healthy exercise, a clean environment, and caring relationships promote health, while junk foods, physical inactivity, a dirty environment, and poor relationships are not good for health. In spite of knowing this, many people persist in unhealthy behaviors that lead to common health problems that plague our world.

Knowing the guidelines for healthy living is not enough by itself. The key is to transform this knowledge into action. It is through action that real change takes place. The challenge to building a healthier lifestyle lies in bridging the gap between knowledge and meaningful action. Bridging this gap is not easy, but it's possible. A healthy lifestyle is eminently achievable, and the rewards it carries are immense.

You can make changes needed to improve your health, and the work involved is worth every ounce of energy at your command. As you follow these guidelines to vibrant living, you will be rewarded. While there is no guarantee to anything in life, these guidelines point the way to optimal health.

Six Simple Suggestions

Following are six simple suggestions to help anyone make change.

1. Keep this guidebook handy so you can refer back to it often when you have any questions.

2. Write the following statement and read it aloud every day: "I choose the power of a healthy lifestyle!" Doing this daily will cement this decision firmly in your mind, and keep it front and center for you.

3. Let your doctor know what you are doing and ask him to support your effort. He or she will probably be delighted with your deci-

sion. If not, try to find a doctor who practices lifestyle medicine in your area to help you. More doctors are beginning to do this as the momentum for lifestyle medicine rapidly gains ground.

4. Find a friend to exercise with you daily. Walking 30 minutes a day is the easiest exercise to adopt, and doing it with a friend makes it fun and effective. You can choose other forms of exercise instead, but whatever you choose, do it with a friend!

5. Start a Healthy Living group in your neighborhood or your church. Developing group support for your new lifestyle will be very helpful to you and to everyone else in the group. Use this book as a basis for discussion to get your group started. Then move on to any other possibilities to help promote healthy lifestyles.

6. Find a nutritionist who can speak to your Healthy Living group once a month if possible. Healthy eating will be a topic of great interest to everyone. You may want to organize healthy potluck meals for your group on a periodic basis. Having a nutritionist to guide, facilitate, and educate at these events is very helpful.

Having adopted a health-empowering lifestyle, don't ever look back and don't ever quit. If you slip, get back on track. Slip-ups happen, but perseverance wins the day. You can make it—Yes, You Can!

Additional Resources to Help Achieve Lifestyle Changes

Today there are abundant resources available for anyone to use in developing a healthy lifestyle. Lifestyle medicine is a relatively new emphasis in mainstream medicine, but it is growing rapidly. In addition to the guidelines in this book, following are a number of good resources to help you on your lifestyle journey.

1. The American College of Lifestyle Medicine (ACLM) is a great resource to learn about physicians who actively promote and teach the principles of lifestyle medicine. It's also a good resource to learn what is new and emerging in lifestyle medicine. Here is its home website: http://www.lifestylemedicine.org/

2. The American College of Preventive Medicine (ACPM) is the professional organization of preventive medicine physicians. The ACPM has a lifestyle medicine initiative and actively works with ACLM, which is one of its academies. Here is the ACPM website: http://www.acpm.org/

3. The American Academy of Family Physicians (AAFP) is the professional organization for family physicians. With over 100,000 members, it is a major force in primary care. Its AIM-HI program (Americans In Motion - Healthy Interventions) is an excellent lifestyle resource for physicians to use in their offices, as well as for individual patients: Here are the websites for the AAFP and its AIM-HI program. http://www.aafp.org/online/en/home.html, http://www.aafp.org/online/en/home/clinical/publichealth/aim/about.html

4. Dr. Joel Fuhrman is a family physician who has written the best-selling book, *Eat to Live*, as well as several other books. He also created the PBS program titled, *3 Steps to Incredible Health*. His nutritionally-oriented practice and research is outstanding. I recommend his books as a good resource for anyone wanting to learn more about a truly healthy way to eat. His website is also a good resource: http://www.drfuhrman.com/

5. Dr. John McDougall is an excellent internist who conducts five-day and ten-day health renewal programs at the McDougall Health and Medical Center in California. As a pioneer in Lifestyle Medicine, he has written numerous books on health and created many out-

standing programs that promote good health. His website offers many resources to help anyone improve their health: http://www.drmcdougall.com/

6. Dr. David Katz is an outstanding internist who founded the Yale University Prevention Research Center as well as the Turn the Tide Foundation, Inc. He has pioneered many lifestyle improvement programs. His new book, *Disease Proof,* provides much practical wisdom about learning the skills of a healthy lifestyle. His website is an excellent resource: http://www.davidkatzmd.com/

7. The Institute of Lifestyle Medicine based at Harvard Medical School is a good resource for physicians. It offers a variety of courses to help physicians upgrade their practices and teaching with regard to lifestyle medicine. Its website is excellent: http://www.instituteoflifestylemedicine.org/index.php

8. Activity Bursts Everywhere (A-B-E) is a good online resource to help people improve their activity levels with quick exercise bursts. Created by Dr. Stephan Esser from Harvard's Institute of Lifestyle Medicine and Dr. David Katz from the Turn the Tide Foundation, this program features short, action-oriented videos that literally show anyone how to exercise more effectively. Here is the website: http://www.abeforfitness.com/

9. Dr. Kenneth Cooper is the legendary physician who launched the Aerobics fitness boom decades ago, and is the founder of the Cooper Clinic in Dallas, Texas. The Cooper Aerobics Health and Wellness website is a good resource for people seeking to learn more about better nutrition and exercise. It offers many programs that provide guidance in these areas. Here is the Cooper Aerobics website: http://www.cooperaerobics.com/Cooper-Clinic.aspx

10. The Centers for Disease Control and Prevention (CDC) offer many programs to help prevent disease and improve health. One of its websites offers the CDC National Prevention Strategy: America's Plan for Better Health and Wellness. This is a good resource to know about: http://www.cdc.gov/features/preventionstrategy/

11. The Environmental Working Group is an excellent organization that promotes a healthy environment for healthier living. Its teams of scientists, engineers, computer experts, lawyers, and policy experts monitor the environment to find solutions that lead to better and healthier products. It's a good resource to consult to learn about food and water safety, as well as a host of commercial cleaning and cosmetic products that might affect health. This website is worth consulting with any questions related to environmental health and safety: http://www.ewg.org/

12. Dr. Jon Kabat-Zinn is world-famous for introducing meditation to millions of people. He founded the Center for Mindfulness in Medicine, Health Care, and Society at the University of Massachusetts Medical School in 1995. Beneficial for stress reduction as well as health enhancement, this center's website is an excellent resource for anyone wanting to learn more about meditation and stress reduction: http://www.umassmed.edu/Content.aspx?id=41252

13. Dr. Barbara Fredrickson is a leading authority on Positive Psychology. Her PEPLab (short for Positive Emotions and Psychophysiology Lab) at the University of North Carolina is an outstanding research center in the field of positive psychology. This website is an excellent resource to learn more about practical applications of positive psychology: http://www.unc.edu/peplab/home.html

14. *Happy Guide* is an ebook by Michael Kinnaird that I recommend highly as a resource. It is an excellent guide to the basics of healthy

living that Michael lays out in easy-to-read fashion. The book is easily downloadable from his website. You can simply click on this link to go to his website featuring his book, and then simply click on the link there to instantly get his book. Here is the link to his website: http://happyguide.co

15. The Vegetarian Resource Group is a good group to know about for those interested in resources for vegetarians or vegans. Following is the link to its website: http://www.vrg.org/

16. *Recipes for Healthy Living* is a good resource found on my website, consisting of many recipes with easy ways to prepare simple wholesome foods, including discussion to highlight points worth emphasizing. Here is a link to the website: http://thepoweroflifestyle.com/free-recipes-for-healthy-living

These are good resources to help anyone wishing to learn more about healthy lifestyles. There are hundreds of additional resources and websites available, but these sites are enough to help anybody get started. The point I wish to emphasize is that you are not isolated in trying to improve your lifestyle. Take advantage of as many of these resources as you wish. Enjoy a well-lived life all of your days!

Lifestyle Stories from Africa

CHAPTER SIXTEEN

Mbakaya's Story

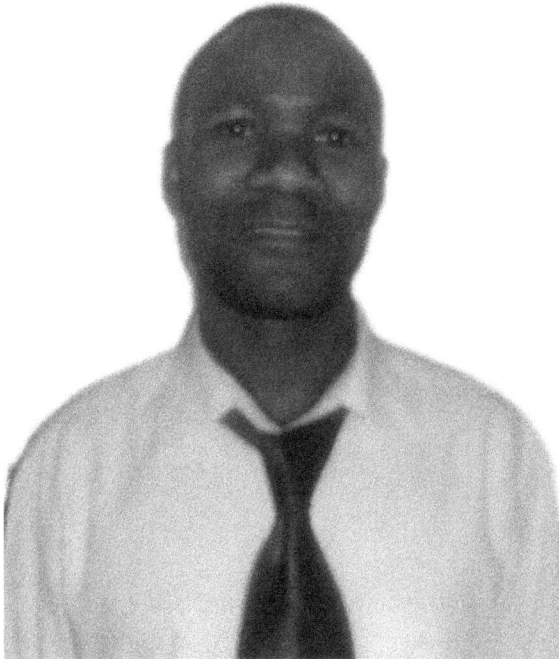

by Balwani C. Mbakaya, BScN, MPH

I am a male who was born in 1977 and grew up in the rural area of Chilumba Malawi. Because of our extended family, my father's pay as a primary school teacher was not enough for the basic needs of the family. Instead, he raised us so we could produce enough food for ourselves as a family, and we ate similar local foods.

My father opted to retire at the age of 50 years so that he could join my mother, who was a housewife, to work in the field. Besides that, he used some of our land to plant several types of fruits (mangos, pawpaws, guavas, bananas, oranges, lemons and others). We used to eat several servings of them per day.

We used to walk long distances to see aunts and uncles, as far as 20 kilometers or more on foot. The primary school I went to for eight years was 1.5 kilometers away from home and I would walk to school two to four times a day. The secondary school I went to was over four kilometers away. I used to walk twice every day to attend classes as a day scholar. Little did I know that this was a healthy lifestyle being practiced at its best.

In 2012 I attended an MPH class taught at Africa University in Zimbabwe. I then reflected on how the kind of lifestyle in which my parents raised our family benefited us. My father is now 81 years but still very strong and working in the field and continuing to eat his local foods. I encourage him to keep doing this.

I have been motivated to adopt a healthier lifestyle since Dr. Dodge's class, especially when I reflect on the benefits I experienced from my upbringing. My father continues to be a living example and a big motivation to practice a healthy lifestyle. I am now 35 years-old and not on any medication with my current lifestyle.

Now I'm engaged in impacting the life of my society where I come from to help people start to practice a healthier lifestyle and enjoy it benefits.

At the family level:

I encourage my father to keep on getting exercise through farming and walking, and to keep eating local foods each time I visit him in the village.

I make sure we eat fruits and vegetables and reduce health sabotaging foods in our daily meals.

My children (a six-year-old first born and five-year-old twins) have been trained to compete in eating more fruits and vegetables by rewarding them with a toy. Now it has become their habit to eat vegetables and carry fruits each time they go to school/nursery.

I have a big yard where we live. I have turned it into a netball and football field with goal posts where we run around and play as a family. The young ones like it so much such that they remind me to buy a new ball as soon as they see that the ball is wearing out.

I have a garden within the yard for fruits and vegetables.

My wife and I managed to buy a piece of land last year that is equivalent to two and a half hectares. It is 23 kilometers away from the town where we live. We plan to plant different fruits this year like bananas, avocados, mangos, oranges, and others. We'll enjoy these as a family, and also sell fruit at a fair price to the community to benefit their health.

At the community level:

I teach at a nursing college with 295 students. Currently I'm teaching non-communicable diseases (NCDs), and I put much emphasis on prevention and healthy lifestyle.

I conduct healthy lifestyle sessions with fellow staff members as a continuing professional development.

We have currently formed a social club with 24 members where we run or play social soccer two to three times a week after knocking off from work, and we want to extend it into becoming a walking and cycling club.

When I want to talk to a member of our staff, instead of using the phone, I now walk to his or her office most of the time.

I am currently conducting a study in our area on healthy lifestyles, and plan to do more studies in this field that has become my major field of interest. I will reach many by sharing my results in publications and through presentations at the national level, as well as locally in hospitals and primary and secondary schools where I live.

I am involved in the curriculum review of nursing education in my country that is due in 2014. I will suggest more input in relation to NCDs and healthy lifestyles so that nursing students become more sensitized to the importance and value of healthy lifestyles in preventing NCDs.

* *

Brief Commentary by Ed Dodge

Mbakaya obtained his Masters of Public Health degree from Africa University in June, 2013. He had previously earned a Bachelor's of Science in Nursing degree as well as a University Certificate in Midwifery from the University of Malawi. He also earned numerous other professional certificates in connection with his work as a nurse and teacher of nurses in Malawi.

Like other MPH students, he learned that the value of the simple rural lifestyle of earlier generations was greater than he had previously realized. He expresses this nicely in his brief autobiography. Unfortunately, today many urbanized educated Africans downplay the lifestyle value of their rural roots. They may romanticize their rural ancestry in other ways, but they believe that modern ways of life are technologically superior and more sophisticated than traditional ways. Because of this, they tend to underestimate the health value of simpler traditional lifestyles.

Recognizing the health value of his parents lifestyle, Mbakaya is finding ways of instilling those values in his children. His family is incorporating wholesome foods and exercise into their lives, while avoiding highly processed foods and sedentary ways of life that seriously undermine health today. They are strengthening family bonds as they do this, which also contributes to the healthier lifestyle they are practicing.

At the community level, Mbakaya teaches the subject of noncommunicable diseases to nursing students. He is already influencing colleagues and students with regard to putting healthy lifestyle measures into practice, doing so in creative ways that are fun for them. He plans to expand these efforts through continuing research as well as public outreach and education.

Mbakaya is convinced of the value of the healthy lifestyle at both a personal and a community level. He is a brilliant young man who is passionate about living, teaching, and modeling the healthy lifestyle. As a top nursing educator in Malawi, he positively influences nursing students there. By virtue of his training, position and personality, he will have a big impact on a new generation of nurses. Through them, and through his community outreach, he will have a substantial impact on the health of Malawians in the future.

CHAPTER SEVENTEEN

Hellen's Story

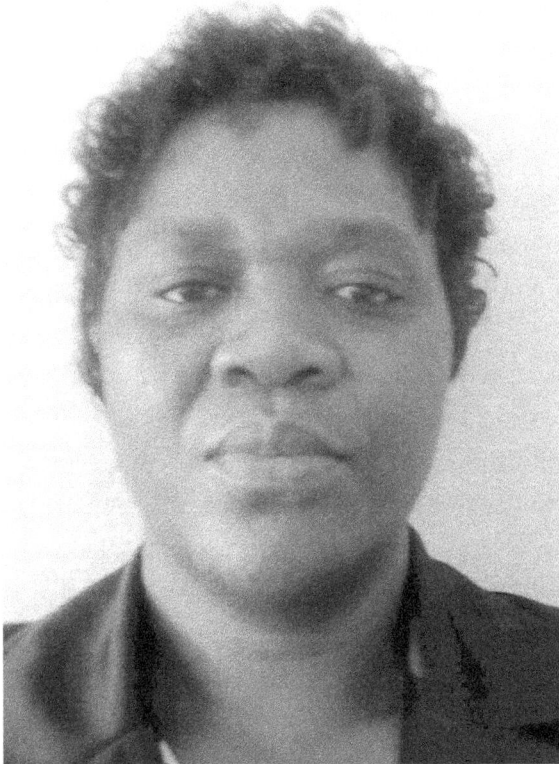

by Hellen Dziwa, BScN, MPH Student

I am a married woman born in Murewa district in the east of Zimbabwe in 1971 as a second born in a family of three children, and my mother's only daughter. I was brought up by my grandparents in Murewa. They were peasant farmers and my grandmother was a village health worker. She taught me a lot about prevention of communicable diseases, especially bilharzia, malaria, scabies and diarrheal diseases. The prevention of these diseases was her job in the village and she would also treat minor ailments including uncomplicated malaria using Chloroquine tablets and doing simple dressings. Because of her knowledge of the complications of the diseases, she would not allow me to bathe or swim with other village girls at the river. As a young girl I used to cheat on her anyway but when she found out, it was a good reason to be beaten up for risking my life. She told me that not preventing diseases that can be prevented created unnecessary expenses for the family when people get sick. Being a young girl then I felt she was being very unfair to me.

As an adolescent girl I transferred to Harare where my aunt raised me until 1995. During the time that my aunt raised me, she would give me information on prevention of communicable diseases —mainly diarrheal and sexually transmitted infections. My aunt was a nurse and would actually explain what happens for one to get the infections. The education I got was mainly to keep me from getting infections as young girl, especially HIV, which was still a mystery to some cultures. Non-communicable diseases were not an issue during that time. When I stayed with my aunt, the traditional diet continued. She grew different vegetables in her garden and taught me how to cook them in a nutritious way. Fruits were not talked about a lot. She used to discourage a lot of salt and sugar but didn't explain why these were not good As a young girl I concluded that it was because she was hypertensive and wanted us to eat the same diet as she did.

I did my primary education in the rural area called Murewa to the east of Harare and my secondary education at Lord Malvern High School in Harare. Staying with my grandmother and my aunt inspired me to work with people who need help, but I was caught between becoming a social worker or a nurse. By the time I had completed my high school, I had made up my mind to be a nurse.

I started nurse's training in 1991 at Nyadiri Mission School of Nursing. I was qualified in 1994 and have been working as a nurse midwife. After training for nursing at Nyadiri Mission hospital in 1994, I joined St Paul's Mission hospital as a qualified nurse and worked there until December 1995 when I got married and decided to join my husband in Mutambara. I have been working at Mutambara since 1996. Since then I have risen through the ranks by undergoing training to improve myself professionally. In 2009 I graduated from Africa University with a Bachelor of Science Degree in Nursing.

After I joined the nursing profession in 1991, I noticed different ways of preventing and treating diseases in the world. Some ways are expensive and some are not. There were fewer ill people when I was a young nurse. Death within the hospital used to be rare but now it's a daily occurrence both in homes and hospitals. As a nurse, I also realized that more emphasis is put on the prevention of communicable diseases than on non-communicable diseases. In my experience there are no funders who give their funds towards non-communicable diseases. I also realized that until there are alarming statistics, no one worries about putting preventive and control measures into place. As a nurse I've seen that it is very expensive to treat diseases instead of preventing them in the first place.

There are many costs that are incurred. For example, when a father has a stroke, hiring a vehicle to take him to the hospital and all the medical bills that follow are expensive. In addition, work days lost to illness as well as the effects of unemployment or eventual death have a major impact on the family, especially the children, who might end up dropping out of school. Since being a nurse I've noticed that most non-communicable diseases are diagnosed only when there are complications requiring a visit to the hospital. In most cases patients are brought in with fatal complications and die or are bedridden.

After completing my first degree in 2009 I went back to Mutambara hospital where more middle-aged or elderly people were brought to the hospital after collapsing in their homes. When I heard about a public health program for this kind of problem, and read about what it did, I decided this was a better approach towards community health. With this knowledge, I realized that if the health system would go the public health way, less people would have to visit hospitals which are now overburdened with both communicable and non-communicable diseases. I decided to join the Africa University Masters in Public Health (MPH) program to equip myself with the knowledge and skills to concentrate on prevention of disease rather than continuously wasting resources on curative services within the health system.

I hope to be an agent for change within my community after obtaining my public health degree. My wish is to work with my church as well as the ministry of health in Zimbabwe, to pay more attention to the prevention of both communicable and non-communicable diseases. I hope to focus on nutrition messages being given to communities to prevent obesity in particular. I will advocate for the information to be taken into the communities to the people rather than waiting to give health education talks to the patients and their relatives when they visit the hospital as I feel this is delayed information.

When I joined the MPH program at Africa University, I thought it was mainly an issue of preventing communicable diseases, but the second semester of my first year changed me. In all the previous courses I was taught what I was supposed to do for others, but during the non-communicable disease course I was given information that helped me change my way of life, especially regarding eating and exercise habits. I realized that if I did not put this information into practice, I was going to suffer from the consequences of non-communicable disease like many close relatives and friends who had died as a result of preventable diseases. I remembered my grandfather who had died of lung cancer. Of course he had been a chain smoker who used to smoke even unprocessed tobacco. I remembered my marriage officer who died of cardiac arrest after surviving a stroke some years before. He had lived a sedentary life, was morbidly obese and did not exercise. I learned that motivation and dedication are needed to live a healthy lifestyle. In these lessons I understood that exercise, good nutrition and good relationships help an individual live a healthy lifestyle.

What I liked most was learning that eating more vegetables and fruits is best, instead of what had always been said before, that is, that meat was the best for one's health. I had given the diet education to eat meat to patients as a nurse, and what I taught other people about diet is what I had lived, though I liked vegetables from my aunt's upbringing. This course now equips me with better knowledge for my work as a public health officer as well as an advocate for healthy eating in my family.

Learning this information helped me to try healthier ways of living. I actually witnessed the impact of a healthy lifestyle within a few months of putting words into practice. When I started the course I was 92 kilograms (202 pounds) with a BMI of 37. By April, my weight was down to 86 kilograms (189 pounds) with my BMI down to 35. Before beginning to put this information into action, I used to feel short of breath when going uphill or upstairs. My dyspnea disappeared after I started to exercise. I chose to walk up and down three flights of hostel stairs for 30 minutes every morning. Evening exercise included walking away from the hostel with classmates who also got motivated by Dr. Dodge. I now feel more energetic than before and can now walk on any terrain without difficulty, as compared to the days before I began this program. I decided to share this information with my husband and two children so they can also benefit. I will teach them by being exemplary in the home, by doing daily exercise and preparing healthy foods for them. I will increase the variety of vegetables in my backyard garden for my family where I used to grow only carrots, beets, and rape and covo greens.

I have plans in place to take the healthy lifestyle to fellow female workers at Mutambara hospital. I feel it would be very selfish if I don't share this good information with them on a social basis, not only in my work. I plan to start a "Forever Healthy" women's club to help prevent obesity and non-communicable diseases among female health workers. I also wish to share information about the healthy lifestyle with my church when I am through with my studies at Africa University. My wish now is to let the community and my family know that the choices we make today about our physical activity and the food we eat have a great impact on our own future health and the health of our children.

* *

Brief Commentary by Ed Dodge

Hellen grew up with an interest in health work because her grandmother and her aunt were both health workers. As she tells us, she herself became a nurse who constantly worked to improve her knowledge and skills. She obtained a nursing certificate in 1993. Later she earned a Bachelor's of Science in Nursing degree at Africa University in 2009, and then enrolled in the Master of Public Health course at Africa University in 2012. In the meantime, she earned numerous other diplomas in nursing, including a Diploma in Midwifery in 2003 from the Bindura School of Midwifery.

Her course at Africa University has had an impact on her thinking about health, and she has begun putting this into practice in her own life. In addition to influencing her own family, she will have a significant impact on her colleagues and her community because of her position as Sister in Charge (equivalent to Director of Nurses) at Mutambara Hospital. Her story shows how the ripple effect of effective education at Africa University can spread to many others.

CHAPTER EIGHTEEN

Innocent's Story

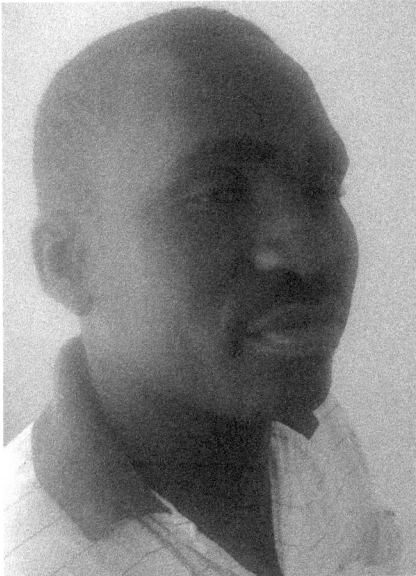

by Innocent Chamusingarevi, BSc in Health Promotion; MPH student

My name is Innocent Chamusingarevi. I am a male who was born on 13 November 1983, the second from last child in our family of five boys and four girls. My birthplace was in Muchiri Village under Chief Makumbe of Buhera District, Manicaland Province, Zimbabwe, which was where I grew up.

Our parents were not employed, so we survived from peasant farming and a small vegetable garden. My mother used to cook home brewed beer to source funds for our primary school fees. I learned about the effects of tobacco smoking and alcohol intake as a young boy. My father used to beat my mother due to the influence of alcohol and dagga smoking. (Note: Dagga is a South African word for marijuana.)

One day when I was ten years old, I had a lot of home brewed beer with sadza. I got drunk that day and as a result, decided not to drink any more alcohol. I still don't drink any alcohol.

We used to eat red meat twice a month and chicken once a month. We were very talented in fishing, so we used to eat fish more than 15 times a month. During adolescence, I learned about the importance of personal hygiene and the effects of tobacco smoking.

I did my primary education at Makumbe Primary School in Buhera district and I went to high school at Makumbe High School in the same district. At my Advanced level I took mathematics, physics and chemistry. I wanted to go into Engineering, but my older brother, who was studying psychology at University of Zimbabwe, applied for me. Instead of Engineering, he enrolled me in the Bachelor of Science program in Health Promotion. Although I didn't choose the field of Health Promotion, I found it interesting. It suits me because I enjoy working with people most of the time.

After completing my degree at the University of Zimbabwe. I joined Medicin Sans Frontieres (Doctors Without Borders) as a trainee health promotion officer. During my internship I worked in the HIV treatment and prevention program. After interning at MSF, I joined Mercy Corps as the district cholera response officer. My duties were community health education and supervision of health promotion activities, as well as distribution of non food items like buckets and soaps.

After working in Mercy Corps, I joined the Zimbabwe Ministry of Health and Child Welfare as District Health Promotion Officer for Buhera district. My work was to provide community health education on communicable and non-communicable diseases. Having found that the prevalence of non-communicable and communicable diseases were on the increase, I decide to enroll in the MPH course at Africa University. My lecturer on non-communicable diseases was Dr. Dodge.

Because of his lectures on the importance of physical activity and a healthy diet. I started a nutrition garden with fifteen types of vegetables, and I began exercising regularly with my wife. She was obese with a Body Mass Index (BMI) of 36.7, while mine was 24.6. In addition to starting a nutrition garden, we began to walk 45 minutes every day. After one month of greater physical activity and eating a diet of wholesome food, fruits and vegetables, my wife's BMI dropped to 35.9. Mine came down to 23.3 from the day we started this lifestyle intervention.

I chose to study the Masters in Public Health course at Africa University so that I could address health issues of common concern. I have experienced the benefits of an improved lifestyle. After completing this course I want to increase community participation in health education and promotion programs. This will help me identify factors that might lead to poor uptake of health care delivery services in the country.

As the District Health Promotion Officer for Buhera District, I have many duties such as writing and producing brochures, running workshops to promote good health, and facilitating the health promotion work of a wide range of organizations. I want to create demand for the control and prevention of non-communicable diseases by increasing awareness of the importance of physical activities and wholesome food, including fruits and vegetables, and by starting behavior change programs for projects such as tobacco smoke cessation among tobacco smokers in my District. My overall goal is to promote access to quality health care, better use of preventive measures, and healthier lifestyles.

* *

Brief Commentary by Ed Dodge

Innocent tells us about his family background and his childhood in the opening paragraphs of his story. He is very frank about the family problems he experienced as he grew up. Yet, he learned from those problems and was able to turn negative experiences into positive outcomes. This says volumes about his character. Even the story of how he accidentally got into the health field says a lot about his ability to adjust and make the best of any situation.

He did well in his Masters course in Public Health at Africa University, applying what he learned to his life and his own family in a very positive way. In addition to the Bachelor of Science degree he earned from the University of Zimbabwe in 2008, he received a Certificate in Clinical and Public Health Research from the Harvard School of Public Health in 2012. His work as the District Health Promotion Officer for the Buhera District will give him a good platform to promote healthy lifestyles. His modeling of the healthy lifestyle he teaches will make him particularly effective in his community.

CHAPTER NINETEEN

Kudzayi's Story

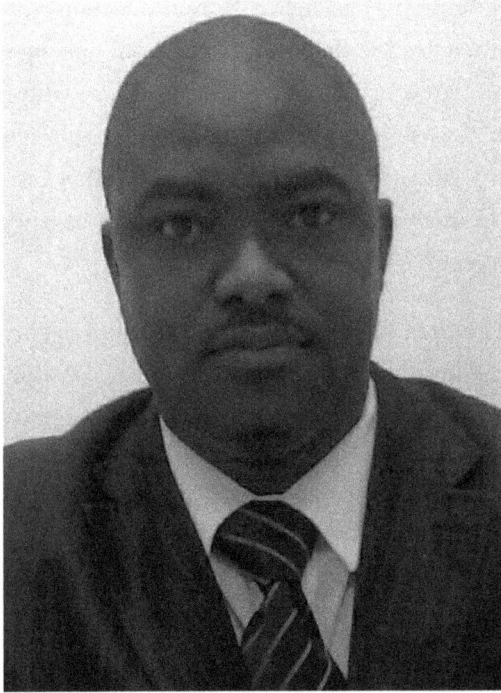

by Kudzayi P. Mukosera, BSc, MBChB, MBA, MPH Student

According to the Bible, after God had created man, he prescribed a healthy diet for him (Genesis 1, vs 29: Then God said: "I shall give you every seed-bearing plant on the face of the whole earth and every tree that has fruit with seed in it. They will be yours for food."). This probably highlights the importance of lifestyle practices in the health of a human being. Various scientific studies have also proven the impact of lifestyle practices on health. The following discussion consists of my personal perspectives and experiences on issues related to the area of lifestyles practices and health.

I was born in July 1976 in Rusape, a small town in the province of Manicaland in Zimbabwe. I arrived into this world as a second son and third born child to a young professional couple who were both civil servants in colonial Rhodesia. My father, who has now passed on, was a teacher who later became a headmaster and then a district education officer. My mother is a nurse who practiced at the local clinic before moving on to the local general hospital. I grew up in a stable religious home with four siblings in the high density township of Tsanzaguru, in the home of relatively affluent parents. Both my parents never drank or smoked. They instilled discipline and social values in all of us. As a result, all five of us have stable, happy, religious marriages and families.

The foundations of lifestyle habits were set from the influence of both parents, older siblings and the social environment. Because neither of my parents drank or smoked, it influenced me not to take up these habits as well. Being raised in a Christian home also set a sound spiritual foundation which has contributed immensely to my own spiritual health. However, there was very little family emphasis on a healthy diet or other healthy lifestyle habits such as exercising. Thus, sticking to a strict healthy diet and an exercise schedule was not part of the daily routine, so these played a lesser role in our lives. My point is that, all in all, the foundations of healthy living were enshrined in our upbringing, including the habits of those who brought us up and the people who were most influential in our lives. Therefore, this is a call to all parents and care givers to set the right standards for your children in terms of lifestyle choices.

I did my primary education at Tsanzaguru Primary School, a local school which my father headed. I proceeded to do my secondary school education at Marondera High School before proceeding to do my 'A' level at Jameson High School, both schools being government boarding schools that offered a Western-influenced way of living and diet. The schools also offered a balanced curriculum of sport and academics and I participated on school teams in basketball, volleyball and soccer. Then I went to the National University of Science and Technology where I obtained my first Bachelor's degree. I then proceeded to the University of Zimbabwe where I studied Medicine and Surgery before obtaining a Masters in Business Administration at the same institution. Most recently, I enrolled in Africa University, a Methodist-related institution where I'm undertaking a Masters in Public Health program at the time of this writing.

Although I have achieved a relatively high standard of education, including learning the advanced tenets of the foundations of healthy living, adhering to healthy lifestyle habits has not been easy. Practicing healthy habits such as exercising and eating a healthy diet has always proved to be a challenge. I have learned that knowledge about good lifestyle practices and lifestyle changes is not enough. There is need for a commitment to change that comes from within. I've also discovered that it's important to have a motivating factor to live a healthy lifestyle. This motivation must be greater than the temptations of unhealthy practices. Without the right healthy lifestyle foundations, an individual will most likely live an unhealthy lifestyle. It takes not only knowledge, but motivation to change and continue to lead a healthy lifestyle.

From personal experiences and discussion with colleagues, I have come up with a personal lifestyle-change model that I believe can bring positive results. This model consists of a series of sequential steps as follows:

Step 1: Awareness—This stage involves one being aware of the need and/or benefits of healthy lifestyle living. It may also involve one becoming aware of the dangers of unhealthy lifestyle habits. Awareness can come from health workers, colleagues, the media, etc.

Step 2: Motivation—For the process of lifestyle-change to start in earnest, one should have a reason or motive to change one's lifestyle.

Motivating factors are related to reward and punishment. If one is already ill with a condition such as diabetes, cutting down on sugar will bring the rewards of better health, whilst on the other hand, a person with a family history of the condition will avoid sugar for fear of developing the diseases ("punishment for unhealthy living").

Step 3: Implementation—This involves an individual actually practicing healthy lifestyle changes, e.g., stopping smoking. This is the most challenging stage as it requires one to have a very high level of discipline and the willpower to overcome temptation. This stage can last from a few minutes to several years. An individual in this stage can either move to step 4 or step 5.

Step 4: Sustained Healthy living—The individual adopts the new healthy lifestyle and continues on this path.

Step 5: Relapse—This stage occurs when an individual fails to sustain healthy habits, perhaps going back to smoking, eating unhealthy foods, failing to exercise regularly, etc. Reasons for this may include giving in to temptation, lack of financial resources to maintain a healthy lifestyle, lack of discipline, lack of time, etc. Many of these reasons mask a loss of motivation. An individual in this stage has to go back to stage two in order to change his or her lifestyle again.

The benefit of this model is that it helps one realize what stage one is in, and therefore take appropriate action to make one's change efforts more successful.

In a medical career spanning eight years, I practiced in various capacities at Parirenyatwa hospital, the biggest, most sophisticated hospital in Zimbabwe. I have also worked at various private institutions as Medical Officer and Chief Medical Officer, and have been a Board member of an Association of Health Insurance companies.

I've learned that the type of job I'm in at any point in my career always influences my lifestyle habits. As an intern I was always under tremendous work pressure and was always moving around to obtain results, submit samples on time, etc. Although this was good for exercise, it meant eating meals on the go, skipping meals, and generally eating an unhealthy diet. Most of my weekends were spent at work which meant I often missed church, compromising my spiritual health. When I became a Medical Officer, consulting patients the whole day made me sedentary and resulted in my gaining weight.

As a medical doctor practicing in Zimbabwe, I also observed a lack of emphasis in the health field on healthy living. A healthy lifestyle may be prescribed for those who have been diagnosed with diseases such as diabetes and hypertension, but lifestyle habits are seldom used as a preventive tool to avoid these diseases in the first place. Moreover, our health insurance companies do not pay for screening and disease-prevention activities, resulting in little attention being paid by doctors and health institutions to this important area as there are no financial benefits to this kind of practice. All in all, the area of lifestyle medicine is highly neglected in the health delivery system in Zimbabwe, despite the immense benefits that can be derived from it.

Having been in clinical practise for eight years in a developing country, I've come to realize that most of our country's health problems can be made worse by poor policies, and at times by bad decision-making by responsible authorities. With a high burden of communicable diseases and a government that was incapable of adequately funding health care, especially during the hyper-inflationary period in Zimbabwe, I personally witnessed the preventable suffering of many people due to a collapsed health system. Although most of the problems experienced were due to lack of finances, others were related to management issues involving slow response to situations, wrong priorities, and a lack of understanding of the importance of community participation and needs.

This realization influenced me to pursue a Masters degree in Public Health with the hope that I can contribute to filling this void. One of the most interesting courses, which has had an immediate impact on me personally and those around me, has been the non-communicable diseases course with its emphasis on a healthy lifestyle. I have been enlightened on the immense benefits of healthy living, not only to the individual but to communities and the country at large.

I learned how the threat of non-communicable diseases is great for developing countries, and most importantly, the immense potential of lifestyle changes to help prevent this threat. From the course I learned about implementing personal lifestyle changes from a whole new perspective and practical viewpoint, and I've already started to practice and reap the benefits of such practices.

For my spiritual health, I am now starting my day with 10 minutes of devotion combined with reading something positive. As a result I have developed a more positive outlook to life, and have even noticed one or two stress wrinkles starting to disappear!

Whereas previously I would come home in the late hours most of the time due to work pressures, I now make sure that no matter how busy my schedule is, I eat dinner with my family. I've also taken over doing homework with the kids. This has increased the bond between me and the kids, and I have been surprised at how much they have matured! My social health has really improved by just implementing this small change.

I have also cut my sugar and carbohydrate intake and have started noticing a reduction in my BMI. Instead of driving most of the time I now walk as often as I can and because of the exercise I feel healthier and more alive than I did before.

Because of these personal experiences and enlightenment, I've also become an advocate for healthy lifestyle habits amongst my family and other spheres of influence. At my current work place, changes have already been made to raise awareness of non-communicable diseases and their link to lifestyle habits. In addition to blood pressure and temperature checks, we are now routinely doing glucometer readings to screen for diabetes, plus height and weight measures for instant determination of Body Mass Index (BMI) on all patients, irrespective of the purpose of the person's visit.

Although I've noted that knowledge alone is not enough for a person to effectively implement lifestyle changes, awareness still remains the first critical step to start the process. As a public health officer, I will advance the healthy lifestyle message in order to combat the threat of lifestyle-linked non-communicable diseases in my country. I'm taking a two-pronged approach that may sound over-ambitious for an individual, but I hope will inspire and guide other public health officers to promote healthy lifestyle habits.

1. Research: Many unhealthy lifestyle habits are promoted by consumerism and commercial interests through advertising and promotions. There is a need for research on the true extent of these practices so concrete evidence can be provided to influence advertising laws in my country. Moreover, corporations have been known to initiate and fund research to produce results tailor-made for their commercial interests, even though they may promote unhealthy lifestyles. Research to counter this is needed. As a Masters in Public Health student, I am seriously considering carrying out research in these areas.

2. Awareness: As I've mentioned above, awareness is the first critical step to lifestyle changes. The process I hope to take starts from educating those individuals that I interact with on a regular basis, such as family members, church members, workmates, patients, etc. The next stage involves mass awareness efforts through mass media. This obviously involves the need for funding. Since the medical insurance industry does not fund for prevention interventions, I hope to raise awareness of the benefits of prevention of disease to health funders and advocate for policy changes in this area.

Once medical insurance companies realize the benefits of cost-cutting due to a healthy membership, I'm confident they will come to the forefront of spreading the healthy lifestyle message, and thus fund mass awareness enterprises.

* *

Brief Commentary by Ed Dodge

Dr. Mukosera came into the MPH class with a very strong health background. (The MBChB degree is a British equivalent to the MD degree in the USA.) His analysis that knowledge by itself is not enough to help people develop healthy lifestyles is on target. Although he had a strong medical background, Dr. Mukosera learned about lifestyle's powerful impact on health while taking the MPH course at Africa University. Like others in his class, he became motivated to make positive changes in his lifestyle and is doing so very effectively.

With his professional qualifications, experience and understanding, he is in an excellent position to help develop the principles of lifestyle medicine in Zimbabwe.

Epilogue

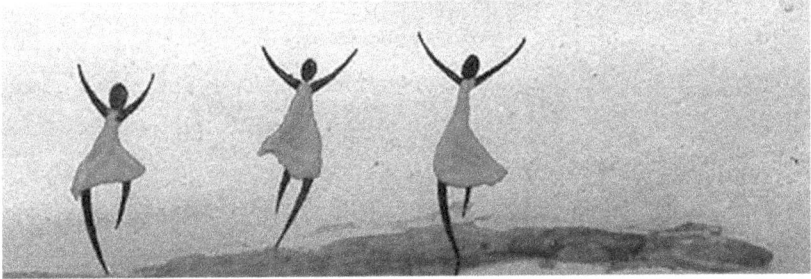

Dear Reader:

Congratulations! Now that you've finished reading this book, you understand why a healthy lifestyle is so rewarding. It's revitalizing at every level of your being, from the cellular to the spiritual. It's no wonder that it lights up your life and lifts your sense of well-being. You also understand now why the movement to healthier lifestyles is taking place around the world.

Leaders across the spectrum in medicine and health care are calling for lifestyle changes as the best answer to the health challenges confronting our country and our world, both at the individual and the societal levels. Being aware of this may help give you added motivation to move toward a healthier lifestyle, but it's unlikely that such knowledge will be enough by itself. You need as many tools as possible to move from knowledge to intelligent action. Every tool you use boosts your chance of success.

In addition to the resources listed for you earlier in this book, here are three more suggestions that may help you. The first is to form a group of individuals who share similar lifestyle goals. We looked at this idea before, but I'm re-emphasizing it here because it is such an important tool. Find two or more other people who want to work on lifestyle improvement and agree to meet weekly to support each other in this adventure. The spirit of mutual support is more important than the size of the group, but three to twelve members is a good size. You will find this to be a powerful help.

The "Wellness Toolkit" mentioned in Appendix B and found on my website is another useful resource. This consists of simple forms designed to support you in each of the four main lifestyle sectors: Nutrition, Physical Activity, Hygiene, and Relationships. Fill in the blanks for one of these sectors every day, taking only a few minutes to give you an ongoing record of your work. This will also be a reminder for you to stay involved, giving you a boost in that area every day.

Each sector is designed to give you this framework of support for 28 days, after which you probably won't need it any longer. You can work in all four sectors at once, or you can work in one area for four weeks and then move to the next sector. Either approach has its pros and cons. Whatever way you choose to do this is fine. (The Wellness Toolkit is available on my website for anyone who wishes to engage in a healthy lifestyle adventure to download freely.)

My third suggestion is to find a Health Coach who can guide you through your lifestyle adventure for the first few months. A certified Health Coach is expert at helping you stay in touch with your inner self and be true to your commitment to yourself. The Health Coach is not likely to be a physician but is someone who has been specifically trained in coaching others to help them achieve their goals. A Health Coach can be a great help to you in your lifestyle adventure. You are not alone in the wilderness trying to improve your lifestyle.

To conclude, remember that no single activity makes or breaks health by itself. It is the overall life pattern that is important. The healthy lifestyle is not complicated. It is eminently achievable, and the rewards it carries are immense.

Even if we as a people applied only the simple priorities of walking 30 minutes daily and eating six servings of fruit and veggies every day, we could dissolve our country's health care crisis in less than a year. Our national health would be so much improved that our disease care system would no longer be in crisis mode. This won't happen because most people haven't caught this vision yet. When they grasp it, we will become a healthier nation.

In the meantime, you can make any changes needed to make your life healthier. The work involved is worth every ounce of effort, but this is not a crash course. Often, baby steps toward your goal prove to be the most effective. There are no guarantees to anything in life, but these guidelines point the way to good health. May you enjoy a life well-lived for all of your days!

APPENDIX A

Chemicals in Our Environment

We are awash in man-made chemicals today. They are everywhere —in our homes, our food, our water, our clothes, our yards, our office buildings, our stores, our streets, our farms, and even in the air we breathe. In the nineteenth century of John Snow's time, such chemicals were rare. The dramatic increase of man-made chemicals in our environment came after 1945, with the invention and commercialization of thousands of petrochemical products after World War II.

The Chemical Abstract Service has registered over 60 million new chemicals since 1956. About 100,000 chemicals are in commercial use in the United States today. They are found in every conceivable niche of our environment and our homes. It is literally impossible to escape them. Many of them are useful, but many have negative long-term effects that are hazardous to the environment and to health. Most of them were not thoroughly tested for safety before being marketed.

Some of the health problems triggered by chemicals include allergic reactions, asthma, chronic lung disease, autoimmune disorders, immune system weakening, neurological disorders, hormonal disorders (due to chemical endocrine disrupters,) learning disorders, bone marrow dysfunction, and various kinds of cancer. This listing is not complete, but it provides an idea of the scope of health problems involved.

Unfortunately, years can elapse before dangers connected to a specific chemical become apparent. Worse yet, many new chemicals are approved for commercial use with little or no safety testing. Although we live in a chemical environment that poses threats to health, industry's position is that chemicals are usable unless proven toxic.

Many health authorities believe that the opposite principle should be followed: Chemicals should be proven safe before they are released for commercial use. To do otherwise makes us all guinea pigs during the long time-lag before adverse health effects such as cancer become apparent. Nature itself has become the subject of a vast global experiment, and it is no exaggeration to say that we are living in the midst of that experiment today.

Concerned Scientists

Two scientists have been particularly outspoken about the hazards posed by the chemicals in our environment. Samuel Epstein, MD, Professor Emeritus of Environmental and Occupational Medicine at the University of Illinois, has led scientific research on this topic for decades. He is the author of over 260 scientific articles and ten books. He has been a consultant to Congress on numerous occasions, and has been a member of key federal agency advisory committees.

Dr. Epstein states: "It is now beyond scientific dispute that environmental and occupational exposures to carcinogens are the primary cause of non-smoking related cancers."[64] He adds, "We are not winning the war against cancer. We are losing the war... while our ability to treat and cure most common cancers has remained virtually unchanged."[65]

Dr. Sandra Steingraber is an award-winning scientist who wrote the

---

64. http://www.huffingtonpost.com/samuel-s-epstein/president-obama-and-the-c_b_435547.html?ref=email_share

65. Samuel S. Epstein, MD. *The Politics of Cancer Revisited*, (Fremont Center, NY: East Ridge Press, 1998).

book, *Living Downstream*, in 1997. The book's subtitle is: *A Scientist's Personal Investigation of Cancer and the Environment*. It is personal because she is a cancer survivor herself. Her book is a wide-ranging investigation of how chemicals have infiltrated every facet of our environment and are implicated in the growing prevalence of cancer in our country. Its central theme is that we are all living downstream when it comes to chemicals and other environmental hazards.

Steingraber's most recent book, *Raising Elijah*, is about bringing up Elijah, her young son, in a world widely contaminated with environmental hazards of all kinds. In spite of its serious subject, it is a delightful book, as Steingraber deftly intertwines stories about their family life with concerns about the environmental threats to their future.

An industrial process called hydrofracturing, or "fracking" for short, poses an environmental hazard that concerns many people today. In this process, wells are drilled about a mile deep. The drills are then turned at right angles to go horizontally through deep shale formations. Millions of gallons of water and highly toxic chemicals are pumped through the shale at high pressure to fracture it. This is done to open gas pockets trapped in the shale so the gas can be used commercially.

Steingraber writes eloquently about the environmental degradation and the threats to human health caused by fracking.[66] It is a threat to major aquifers and other water resources. Tremendous volumes of water and toxic chemicals are left in deep underground strata forever. If wells or pipelines traversing aquifers ever blowout, a toxic brew could contaminate precious water resources forever. As Steingraber says, it is madness to consider violating our environment in these ways. The fact that we are doing it anyway shows how deeply addicted our society is to fossil fuels.

---

66. Sandra Steingraber, PhD. *Raising Elijah*, (Philadelphia, PA: Da Capo Press, 2011), pp 270-284.

The Precautionary Principle

Better solutions are possible! In January, 1998, an international group of people met to discuss ways of protecting us from environmental hazards. The group included top scientists, physicians, lawyers, governmental officials, and many others. After three days of meetings, they issued a statement called the "Wingspread Statement," named for Frank Lloyd Wright's Wingspread house in Racine, Wisconsin where the conference was held.[67]

The essence of this statement is that, because of compelling evidence of damage to humans and the environment due to the release and use of toxic substances, it is time to adopt a precautionary approach to such activities. This principle, called the Precautionary Principle, places responsibility on advocates of any potentially hazardous activity to take precautions early on instead of waiting until after-the-fact proof of serious harm to health.

The Precautionary Principle is important today because of widespread chemical pollution. Some responsible organizations have adopted this principle, but many have not. Until they do, each of us must be wise in our personal practices.

Industry Profits May Override Health Concerns

Marion Nestle, Professor of Nutrition, Food Studies, and Public Health at New York University, has written about problems with food politics. Her PhD in molecular biology and MPH in public health nutrition give her a voice in nutrition that is highly respected. She was senior nutrition policy advisor in the Department of Health and Human Services from 1986-88, as well as managing editor of the 1988 Surgeon General's Report on Nutrition and Health.

---

67. Sandra Steingraber, PhD. *Living Downstream*, (New York, NY: Vantage Books, 1998) p. 284.

In her book, *What to Eat,* Nestle notes that marketing to children is big business for the food companies involved. Research shows that "marketing enormously influences kids' choices of brands and food categories, particularly of the heavily advertised breakfast cereals, soft drinks, candy, snacks, and fast foods."[68] Johnnie likes sugary treats because they're sweet, but he was set up to beg for them by all the advertising he's seen on TV.

Nestle cites estimates that marketers spend about fifteen billion dollars a year to promote products aimed at children. She says that food marketing to kids is done with "undisguised cynicism." Food companies market foods for their bottom line, not out of any concern for health. If kids become obese from eating too much of the junk foods being advertised, the food producers disclaim any responsibility, saying it's the job of parents to monitor the food intake of their children. [69]

Besides huge advertising budgets, large corporations exert major lobbying efforts to influence governmental agencies in their favor. Marion Nestle cites an example regarding meat. By 1961, the American Heart Association advised eating less saturated fat and meat. In 1977, the government issued similar advice. Protests from the beef industry "were immediate and vehement." As a result, the clear advice to "Eat less meat" was eventually changed to a vague, "Limit use of animal fats."[70]

Nestle is not against eating meat. She specifically says that a small amount of meat in the diet is fine. Still, after noting the ways in which the meat industry has influenced governmental actions for many years, Nestle concludes that the US dietary meat guideline is a prime example of "food politics in action." Politics by the meat industry puts profits above public health. In addition to affecting diet guidelines, the result of such politics

68. Marion Nestle. *What to Eat,* (New York, NY. North Point Press, 2006) p 373.

69. Ibid., p 377.

70. Ibid., p 149.

can be "pervasive risks to the safety of the food supply."[71]

Concentrated Animal Feeding Operations (CAFOs)

There is another way in which the meat industry presents significant public health hazards. CAFOs is the acronym used for Concentrated Animal Feeding Operations. The most familiar of these are large feedlots that feed hundreds of cattle in relatively confined spaces. In a similar way, large pig barns and poultry barns house and feed thousands of animals in confined spaces. The great majority of animals raised for meat in the United States spend most of their lives in CAFOs.

There are many public health concerns about these operations, including animal health, manure management, air quality, and water quality issues. The EPA has issued rules to cope with the environmental problems involved, but it is an ongoing challenge. One of the largest environmental spills in US history occurred when a huge CAFO retaining lagoon ruptured in 1996, releasing nearly 26 million gallons into the New River in North Carolina. The spill killed 10 million fish and was responsible for outbreaks of human skin eruptions and other health problems. [72]

Agricultural subsidies are another factor that distort food choices. Originally intended to help family farmers, large agri-business gets most of the benefits of these subsidies today. They lobby Congress heavily to keep it that way. The result is that field corn, soybeans, wheat, beef, and dairy products are subsidized. Organic farming gets few or no subsidies. That's a major reason why junk foods are more affordable than healthy foods.

---

71. Ibid., p 164.

72. http://en.wikipedia.org/wiki/Concentrated_Animal_Feeding_Operations

Genetically Modified Foods

Genetically modified foods (GM foods) are relevant here for several reasons. Genetic manipulation is a way of combining genes from different species that cannot be done by any natural process. It is a form of genetic pollution, and we don't know the long-term consequences. Results of feeding GM foods to various kinds of animals are not reassuring, and Monsanto has not been up-front about its research, which is not reassuring either.

Soybeans grown in the United States are genetically altered to make them resistant to Roundup. This herbicide, with the active ingredient, glyphosate, is produced by Monsanto to kill most weeds. Heavy use of Roundup has created resistant super-weeds, and the amount of glyphosate sprayed on fields has grown significantly. GM crops and fields are increasingly saturated with this herbicide. Despite denials by Monsanto, glyphosate is considered a health hazard.[73]

Aside from these pollution issues, Monsanto furiously lobbies Congress and the FDA to fend off any labeling requirement for GM foods. It persuaded the FDA that GM foods are "substantially equivalent" to their conventional counterparts, which is not true. The phrase, "substantially equivalent" is scientific nonsense. The genetic and biologic makeup of these kinds of plants is significantly different. The fact that Monsanto has unique patents on their GM seeds is clear evidence of this.

Why does Monsanto work so hard to keep GM foods from being labeled? Clearly, Monsanto does not want us to know what foods have GM ingredients in them. This is an affront to the public, because we should be able to know what we're eating. The food industry estimates that over 70 percent of processed foods have GM food ingredients in them. Since we don't know which foods are involved, the best way to avoid GM foods is

---

73. http://www.sourcewatch.org/index.php?title=Monsanto_and_the_Roundup_Ready_Controversy

to avoid processed foods.

The food industry is not the only one that uses politics to further its own interests. In *The Politics of Cancer Revisited*, Dr. Epstein goes into detail about the way assorted industries have gone to great lengths to deny or obscure any possible relationship between cancer and their industry. After decades of careful research, he says that cancer is often preventable, and that the hidden political factors that block prevention must be recognized.[74]

Political manipulation often makes health issues difficult to resolve. Community efforts to improve public health require cooperative commitment from all parties involved. When businesses and industries advance their own financial interests to the detriment of the public interest, it becomes harder for individuals to improve their personal health.

Still, there is much that individuals can do to safeguard or advance their own health despite adverse commercial and industrial pressures. In addition to steps outlined in previous chapters of this book, concerned citizens working together in the public interest can accomplish much. Finally, never forget the power of the pocketbook. Businesses of all kinds pay more attention to the bottom line than any other factor. If we don't buy their products, they will be motivated to change!

---

74. Samuel S. Epstein, MD. *The Politics of Cancer Revisited*, (Fremont Center, NY: East Ridge Press, 1998).

The Wellness Toolkit — Practicing The Power of Lifestyle

Introduction: *This toolkit is designed to help you begin applying practical guidelines for healthy living. It's divided into four sections to match four major lifestyle principles. Focusing on a single goal in each section makes putting these lifestyle changes into practice as easy as possible. Mapping out the first four weeks of lifestyle change in this way helps you get started, and will empower you to continue on your own.*

The full toolkit is found on my website as a free download for anyone interested. Here I simply describe features of the Wellness Toolkit that will help you put what you've learned in this book into practice. In order to begin this health adventure, go to this page: www.thepoweroflifestyle.com/wellness-toolkit. Taking advantage of this free service will offer you great benefits.

Here are the lifestyle areas covered in the toolkit:

A. Nutrition

The key objective in this section is to enjoy six servings of vegetables and fruits daily. This is such a crucial aspect of good nutrition that it deserves your full attention as you begin applying the power of good nutrition in your life. Success in meeting this objective will improve your health more quickly and effectively than you think possible. The daily nudge provided by this playful, fill-in-the-blanks, healthy eating calendar will give you a powerful boost to improved vitality.

B. Physical Activity

The key objective in this section is for you to enjoy a thirty-minute walk six days a week for four weeks. To keep track of your walking time and the number of steps you take each day, you will need only a watch and a simple pedometer to count your steps. Writing these two things down on your activity calendar every day will help you put your good intentions into action and give a great boost to a healthier you.

C. Hygiene

Your key objective for this section is to spend ten minutes daily working on good dental hygiene. This may surprise you. Why dental hygiene? It's more important to overall health than most people realize. Practically speaking, it can save you a great deal of long-term grief. Yet, it's often neglected or done superficially. Tooth decay is the most common chronic disease in children, affecting one out of five children. Adults fare no better. Nearly a fourth of adults between the ages of 20-64 have untreated cavities, while about a fourth of those over the age of 64 have lost all of their teeth due to lack of care.

Almost half of younger adults have inflamed gums (gingivitis). Tooth decay and gingivitis are caused by dental plaque that develops about 30 minutes after eating. Plaque is a combination of bacteria, food debris, and saliva that coats the teeth. If left uncleaned, it begins eroding tooth enamel, which is the start of dental caries. Frequent snacking, sugary drinks and failure to brush teeth all contribute to this destructive process. According to the American Dental Association, only 57 percent of women and 49 percent of men brush their teeth at least twice a day. Half of all adults don't floss their teeth daily, and about a fifth of them never floss. Clearly, there is a serious need for better dental hygiene in America.

A good dental routine takes a few minutes after each meal. This time investment can help safeguard health and prevent much pain and cost down the road. To keep track, simply fill in the blank as to how often you brush your teeth and floss your teeth each day. (Aim to brush your teeth at least twice a day and floss them at least once a day.) Strengthening your dental cleaning routine provides an excellent boost to your overall health.

D. Relationships

Caring relationships are more important to health than many people realize. This includes caring for yourself as well as those around you. The key goal here is to focus on dedicating ten minutes to quiet time each day. This time of connecting with your inner self has great value. I call this *Quiet Time* because this simple phrase carries no preformed associations, and because it's an accurate description of this time.

To engage in ten minutes of quiet time most effectively, choose a time when you can sit quietly at a fairly consistent time of day. Being consistent with your quiet time helps you make it a regular part of your life. Even then, it is not ironclad. It's all right to have your quiet time at a different time than usual when necessary. It's also OK to devote more than ten minutes to your quiet time, or have it more often than once a day.

When you enter your quiet time, it works best to sit quietly with your eyes closed, without any agenda on your mind. It can be helpful to focus on a word like *love* or *peace*. At the conclusion of your *Quiet Time*, as you are beginning to re-focus on the outer world, take an extra moment to think about three blessings that you experienced in the preceding twenty-four hours. They can be anything from contact with a friend or family member to enjoyment of a food, a beautiful object, or a special moment of experience. Writing down a few blessings every day will do wonders for both you and those around you.

Next Steps

When you complete the "Wellness Toolkit" you will have gained much inner strength and you will be well positioned to continue your health adventure. There are several ways you can do this.

1. If you're not already in a wellness-oriented group, you can form a small group of friends to continue doing this together. I recommend this strongly. The value of family and friends working on this kind of self-improvement project is beyond great. Being accountable to a group provides strong motivation, while the reinforcement each person gives and receives in a group like this is very powerful. Plan to meet weekly if possible.

2. Another good option is to get in touch with a professional Health Coach who is specifically trained to guide clients in ways to achieve their goals. The coach does not set the goals for you. You set your own goals. The Health Coach simply helps you find the ways and means to reach your goals. The Health Coach is a valuable helper and guide in your endeavor.

3. You can continue your health journey on your own if you wish. If you go this route, support yourself with as many tools as you can and use them frequently. If possible, become a member of your local YMCA or other similar organizations to take advantage of their many health-oriented programs. Although you're on your own, enlisting help from others and enrolling in supportive programs have great value.

The final word? Congratulations! You have come a long way in discovering the power of lifestyle. Keep it up!

About Dr. Ed Dodge

Born in 1936, Ed Dodge grew up as a missionary kid in Angola, Africa. Some of his adventures included living in the wilds of northern Angola, hunting for wild game, and traveling across many poorly charted areas of Africa. He first visited Zimbabwe at age 12 when his parents drove across Africa with their four children to attend a missionary conference.

He graduated from the Indiana University School of Medicine with his MD degree in 1962. Earning the Master of Public Health degree at Johns Hopkins University School of Public Health in 1967, he became an Assistant Professor at the Public Health College in Gondar, Ethiopia for two years. When he returned to the United States, much of his career was spent in Florida where he directed a local health department for a few years and was a family physician for many years. He also served as Courtesy Clinical Associate Professor in the Department of Community Health and Family Medicine at the University of Florida.

After retiring in 1996, Dr. Dodge made numerous Volunteer-in-Mission trips to Zimbabwe over a number of years. In 2010, he was appointed as a volunteer Visiting Adjunct Professor at Africa University in Zimbabwe, teaching in the Master of Public Health program for one semester each year since then. His years of experience in clinical and public health in both Africa and the USA have given him a broad perspective of health challenges in both the developing and the developed world. Through his experiences, he grew to understand the great value of embracing the whole person, body, mind and spirit.

Realizing from a lifetime of caring for patients that most people wish to be healthy, Dr. Dodge was motivated to write about the joys and strengths of holistic health that almost anyone can achieve. *Be Healthy* is the end result of three years of research and a lifetime of learning.

Dr. Dodge has three children and ten grandchildren. He and his wife live in San Antonio, Texas when he is not doing volunteer work or teaching in Africa.

Find out more at
ThePowerofLifestyle.com

The Foundation for Healthy Africa

The Foundation for Healthy Africa was established to promote healthy lifestyles in Africa in response to the developing crisis of non-communicable diseases (NCDs) in Africa. "Western" diseases such as diabetes, obesity, hypertension, heart disease, and stroke were rare in Africa until recent decades. They are now striking hard in many countries in Africa, where officials are ill-prepared to cope with them because available resources are primarily focused on communicable diseases that still remain serious threats to health and well-being. Major health organizations such as the World Health Organization (WHO) and the Centers for Disease Control (CDC) in the USA advise promoting healthy lifestyles as the best answer to combating NCDs. Both WHO and the CDC state that 75 to 80 percent of many NCDs are preventable. Healthy lifestyles are the most effective way to accomplish this. Recognizing this, the Faculty of Health Sciences at Africa University is establishing a Center for Lifestyle Excellence. Its vision is to:

- Conduct research to document lifestyle characteristics prevalent in Africa today;

- Determine lifestyle modifications that will most effectively support healthy lifestyles in Africa;

- Determine effective ways of promoting healthy lifestyles that will work well in Africa;

- Teach students the principles of lifestyle excellence so they in turn can teach and model healthy lifestyles;

- Teach the principles of healthy living in African schools, churches, and other community organizations.

The Foundation for Healthy Africa will fund projects designed to promote healthy lifestyles in Africa, including the Africa Center for Lifestyle Excellence proposed as a research and educational center at Africa University. It will also fund a limited number of graduate scholarships designed to strengthen research and promotion of Healthy Lifestyles.

To learn more visit
FoundationforHealthyAfrica.org

www.ingramcontent.com/pod-product-compliance
Lightning Source LLC
Chambersburg PA
CBHW032104280326
41933CB00009B/754